TABLE OF CONTENTS

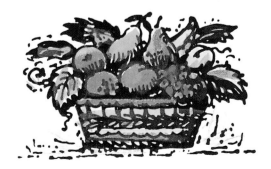

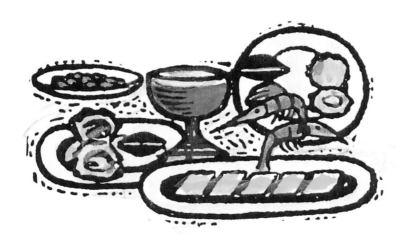

Your diet is an important part of your treatment for cancer. Eating the right kinds of foods during your treatment can help you feel better and stay stronger.

The National Cancer Institute (NCI) has prepared this booklet to help you learn more about your diet needs and how to manage eating problems. Eating well is extra important when your body is fighting disease.

This booklet is mainly for patients who are still receiving cancer treatment. However, it may also be useful after you finish treatment. Pick it up any time you find that eating well is a challenge.

You may not want to read all of this booklet at one sitting. Flip through it to see which sections are useful to you now. Save it so that you can refer to other sections as needed.

Your registered dietitian, doctor, and nurse are your best sources of information about your diet. The information in this booklet will add to their advice. Feel free to ask them for help and to talk with them about changes in your diet. Ask them to explain or repeat anything that is not clear.

At the end of this booklet, you will find information about other free NCI publications about cancer, its treatment, and coping with the illness. We have also listed several resources, reference books, and cookbooks you may find helpful, including the NCI-supported Cancer Information Service (CIS) (1-800-4-CANCER). The CIS provides information about cancer, cancer treatment, research studies, and living with cancer to patients, their families, health professionals, and the general public.

We hope this resource will help you eat better and feel better during and following your cancer treatment.

EATING
WELL DURING CANCER TREATMENT

A nutritious diet is always vital for your body to work at its best. Good nutrition is even more important for people with cancer. Why?

- Patients who eat well during their treatment are better able to cope with the side effects of treatment. Patients who eat well may even be able to handle a higher dose of certain treatments.

- A healthy diet can help keep up your strength, prevent body tissues from breaking down, and rebuild tissues that cancer treatment may harm.

- When you are unable to eat enough food or the right kind of food, your body uses stored nutrients as a source of energy. As a result, your natural defenses are weaker and your body cannot fight infection as well. Yet, this defense system is especially important to you now, because cancer patients are often at risk of getting an infection.

What Kinds of Food Do I Need?

A good rule to follow is to eat a variety of different foods every day. No one food or group of foods contains all of the nutrients you need. A diet to keep your body strong will include daily servings from these food groups:

Fruits and Vegetables: Raw or cooked vegetables, fruits, and fruit juices provide certain vitamins (such as A and C) and minerals the body needs.

Protein Foods: Protein helps your body heal itself and fight infection. Meat, fish, poultry, eggs, and cheese give you protein as well as many vitamins and minerals.

Grains: Grains, such as bread, pasta, and cereals, provide a variety of carbohydrates and B vitamins. Carbohydrates provide a good source of energy, which the body needs to function well.

Dairy Foods: Milk and other dairy products provide protein and many vitamins and are the best source of calcium.

The chart on page 4, "Eat a Variety of Foods Each Day," shows recommended guidelines for a healthful diet. Below is a sample menu that follows these guidelines.

While these standards are a good goal, you also need to listen to your body. If you get nauseous eating fruits but can keep protein foods down, feel free to eat more than 2 servings of protein and less than 4 fruits. Anything you eat will be a plus in helping you get enough calories and maintain your weight.

Sample Menu for Good Nutrition

The following sample menu supplies the minimum number of servings from each food group. If you need to include extra calories in your diet, you may add more servings and include snacks, appetizers, desserts, and drinks from the lists on pages 24 and 25.

Breakfast

½ cup cooked cereal
1 cup milk
½ cup fruit or juice
Beverage
1 slice toast with 1 pat
    margarine or butter

Lunch

Sandwich:
    2 slices bread
    2-3 oz. meat/fish/poultry
    1 tsp. mayonnaise
    1 slice each lettuce, tomato
    1 piece fruit

Dinner

2-3 oz. meat/fish/poultry
½ cup vegetable
½ cup grain product
    (e.g., pasta)
1 slice bread
1 pat margarine or butter
1 cup milk

Snack

½ sandwich:
1 oz. meat/fish/poultry
    1 slice bread
    lettuce
½ cup fruit
½ cup raw vegetables

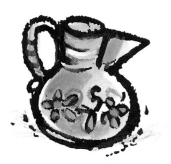

Figure 1. EAT A VARIETY OF FOODS EACH DAY

Food Group	Suggested Daily Servings	What Counts as a Serving?
Breads, Cereals, and Other Grain Products Whole-grain Enriched	6 servings from entire group (include several servings of whole-grain products daily).	■ 1 slice of bread ■ ½ hamburger bun or English muffin ■ a small roll, biscuit, or muffin ■ 3 to 4 small or 2 large crackers ■ ½ cup cooked cereal, rice, or pasta ■ 1 ounce of ready-to-eat breakfast cereals
Fats, Sweets, and Alcoholic Beverages	Avoid too many fats and sweets. If you drink alcoholic beverages, do so in moderation.	
Fruits Citrus, melon, berries Other fruits	2 servings from entire group	■ a whole fruit such as medium apple, banana, or orange ■ a grapefruit half ■ a melon wedge ■ ¾ cup of juice ■ ½ cup of berries ■ ½ cup cooked or canned fruit ■ ¼ cup dried fruit

Can Good Nutrition Treat Cancer?

Doctors know that patients who eat well during cancer treatment are better able to cope with treatment side effects. *However, there is no evidence that any kind of diet or food can either cure or stop it from coming back.* In fact, some diets may be harmful, especially those that don't include a wide variety of foods. There is also no evidence that diet supplements, such as vitamin or mineral pills, can cure cancer or stop it from coming back.

The NCI strongly urges you to eat nutritious foods and follow the treatment program prescribed by a doctor who uses accepted and proven methods or treatment. People who depend on unproven treatments may lose valuable treatment time and reduce their

	Figure 1. Continued	
Food Group	**Suggested Daily Servings**	**What Counts as a Serving?**
Vegetables Dark-green leafy Deep-yellow Dry beans and peas (legumes) Starchy Other vegetables	3 servings from entire group (include all types regularly; use dark-green leafy vegetables and dry beans and peas severals times a week).	■ ½ cup of cooked vegetables ■ ½ cup of chopped raw vegtables ■ 1 cup of leafy raw vegtables, such as lettuce or spinach
Meat, Poultry, Fish, and Alternates (eggs, dry beans and peas, nuts, and seeds)	2 servings from entire group	Amounts should total 5 to 7 ounces of cooked lean meat, poultry, or fish a day. Count 1 egg, ½ cup cooked beans, or 2 tablespoons peanut butter as 1 ounce of meat.
Milk, Cheese, and Yogurt	2 servings from entire group (3 servings for women who are pregnant or breastfeeding and for teens; 4 servings for teens who are pregnant or breastfeeding).	■ 1 cup of milk ■ 8 ounces of yogurt ■ 1½ ounces of natural cheese ■ 2 ounces of process cheese

Source: USDA "Preparing Foods and Planning Menus Using the Dietary Guidelines."

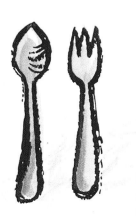

chances of controlling cancer and getting well.

The NCI also recommends that you ask your doctor or nutritionist before taking any vitamins or mineral supplements. Too much of some vitamins or minerals can be just as dangerous as too little. Large doses of some vitamins may even stop your cancer treatment from working the way it should. To avoid problems, don't take these products on your own. Follow your doctor's directions for safe results.

MANAGING EATING PROBLEMS DURING TREATMENT

All the usual methods of treating cancer—surgery, radiation therapy, chemotherapy, and biological therapy (sometimes called immunotherapy)—have to be very strong. Although treatments target the cancer cells in your body, they sometimes can damage normal, healthy cells at the same time. This may produce unpleasant side effects that cause eating problems (see chart "How Cancer Treatments Can Affect Eating"). The side effects may affect your ability or desire to eat.

Side effects of cancer treatment vary from patient to patient. The part of the body being treated, length of treatment, and the dose of treatment also affect whether side effects will occur. Ask your doctor about how your treatment may affect you.

The good news is that only about one-third of cancer patients have side effects during treatment, and

Figure 2. HOW CANCER TREATMENTS CAN AFFECT EATING

Cancer Treatment	How It Can Affect Eating	What Sometimes Happens: Side Effects
Surgery	Increases the need for good nutrition by putting stress on the body. May stop parts of the body that are needed for eating from working properly, such as stomach, mouth, throat. May also make them sore.	Before surgery, a high-protein, high-calorie diet may be prescribed if a patient is underweight or weak. After surgery, some patients may not resume normal eating at first. They may receive nutrients: ■ Through a needle in their vein (IV or intravenous feeding). ■ Through a tube in their nose or stomach. ■ By drinking clear liquids (see pages 28-29). ■ By following a full-liquid diet (see pages 30-31).
Radiation Therapy	May harm parts of the body as it damages cancer cells.	Treatment of head, neck, or chest may cause: ■ Dry mouth. ■ Sore mouth. ■ Sore throat. ■ Change in taste of food. ■ Dental problems.

most side effects go away when treatment ends. Your doctor will try to plan a treatment that keeps side effects down.

Cancer treatment may also affect your eating in another way. When some people are upset, worried, or afraid they may have eating problems. Losing your appetite and nausea are two normal responses to feeling nervous or fearful. Such problems should only last a short time.

While you are in the hospital, your health care team can help you plan your diet. They can also help you solve your physical or emotional eating problems. Feel free to talk to them if problems arise during your recovery as well. Ask them what has worked for their other patients.

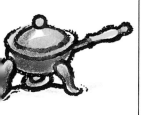

Cancer Treatment	How It Can Affect Eating	What Sometimes Happens: Side Effects
Radiation Therapy (continued)		Treatment of stomach may cause: ■ Nausea. ■ Vomiting. ■ Diarrhea.
Chemotherapy	May harm parts of the body needed for eating as it destroys cancer cells.	■ Nausea and vomiting. ■ Loss of appetite. ■ Diarrhea. ■ Constipation. ■ Sore mouth or throat. ■ Weight gain. ■ Change in taste of food.
Biological Therapy (sometimes called Immuno-therapy)	Not known.	■ Nausea and vomiting. ■ Diarrhea. ■ Sore mouth. ■ Severe weight loss (anorexia). ■ Dry mouth. ■ Change in taste of food.

Figure 2. Continued

Don't be afraid to give food a chance. Not everyone has problems with eating during cancer treatment. Even those who have eating problems have days when eating is a pleasure.

Coping With Side Effects

This section offers practical hints for coping with treatment side effects that may affect your eating.

These suggestions have helped other patients manage eating problems that can be frustrating to handle. Try all the ideas to find what works best for you. Share your needs and concerns with your family and friends, particularly those who prepare meals for you. Let them know that you appreciate their support as you work to take control of eating problems.

Loss of Appetite

Loss of appetite or poor appetite is one of the most common problems that occurs with cancer and its treatment. Many things affect appetite, including feeling sick (having nausea, vomiting) and being upset or depressed about having cancer. A person who has these feelings, whether physical or emotional, may not be interested in eating.

You may find the following suggestions helpful in making mealtimes more relaxed so that you will feel more like eating.

- Stay calm, especially at mealtimes. Don't hurry your meals.

- Involve yourself in as many normal activities as possible. But, if you feel uneasy and do not want to take part, don't force yourself.

- Try changing the time, place, and surroundings of meals. A candlelight dinner can make mealtime more appealing. Set a colorful table. Listen to soft music while eating. Eat with others or watch your favorite TV program while you eat.

- Eat whenever you are hungry. You do not need to eat just three main meals a day. Several smaller meals throughout the day may be even better.
- Add variety to your menu. Try some of the recipes in the "Recipes for Better Nutrition During Cancer Treatment" section at the back of this book.
- Eat food often during the day, even at bedtime. Have healthy snacks handy. Taking just a few bites of the right foods or sips of the right liquids every hour or so can help you get more protein and calories. You can find ideas for preparing healthy snacks on page 20.

Sore Mouth or Throat

Mouth sores, tender gums, and a sore throat or esophagus often result from radiation therapy, anticancer drugs, and infection. If you have a sore mouth or gums, see your doctor to be sure the soreness is a treatment side effect and not an unrelated dental problem. The doctor may be able to give you medicine that will control mouth and throat pain. Your dentist also can give you tips for care of your mouth.

Certain foods will irritate an already tender mouth and make chewing and swallowing difficult. By carefully choosing the foods you eat and by taking good care of your mouth, you can usually make eating easier. Here are some suggestions that may help:

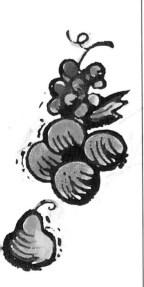

- Try soft foods that are easy to chew and swallow such as:
  —Milkshakes.
  —Bananas, applesauce, and other soft fruits.
  —Peach, pear, and apricot nectars.
  —Watermelon.
  —Cottage cheese.
  —Mashed potatoes, macaroni and cheese.
  —Custards, puddings, and gelatin.

—Scrambled eggs.
—Oatmeal or other cooked cereals.
—Pureed or mashed vegetables such as peas and carrots.
—Pureed meats.
—Liquids.

- Cook foods until they are soft and tender.

- Cut foods into small pieces.

- Mix food with butter, thin gravies, and sauces to make it easier to swallow.

- Use a blender or food processor to puree your food.

- Use a straw to drink liquids.

- Try foods cold or at room temperature. Hot and warm foods can irritate a tender mouth and throat.

- Avoid foods that can irritate your mouth, such as:
  —Citrus fruit or juice such as oranges, grapefruits, tangerines.
  —Spicy or salty foods.
  —Rough, coarse, or dry foods such as raw vegetables, granola, toast.

- If swallowing is hard, tilting your head back or moving it forward may help.

- If your teeth and gums are sore, your dentist may be able to recommend a special product for cleaning your teeth.

- Rinse your mouth with water often to remove food and bacteria and to promote healing.

- Ask your doctor about anesthetic lozenges and sprays that can numb the mouth and throat long enough for you to eat meals.

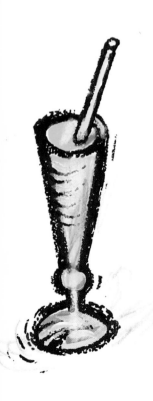

Changed Sense of Taste

Your sense of taste may change. Chemotherapy, radiation therapy, or the cancer itself may cause this problem. Sometimes called mouth blindness or taste blindness, it may cause a change in the way foods taste. Some patients complain of a bitter, metallic taste, especially when eating meat or other protein foods. Patients also may find that many foods have less taste. This is usually a short-term problem.

Each person's taste may be affected differently. You will need to learn which, if any, foods taste different to you. Depending on how your taste has been affected, some of the following ideas for improving flavor may work better than others. In addition, visit your dentist to check for dental problems that may affect food's taste. You can also ask your dentist about special mouthwashes and good mouth care.

Here are some tips to help your food taste better. *(If you also have a sore mouth, sore gums, or a sore throat, talk to your doctor or registered dietitian. They can suggest ways to improve the taste of your food without hurting the sore areas.)*

- Choose and prepare foods that look and smell good to you.
- If red meat (such as beef) tastes strange, use chicken, turkey, eggs, dairy products, or fish that doesn't have a strong smell instead.
- Help the flavor of meat, chicken, or fish by marinating it in sweet fruit juices, sweet wine, Italian dressing, or sweet-and-sour sauce.
- Try using small amounts of flavorful seasonings such as basil, oregano, or rosemary.
- Try tart foods such as oranges or lemonade that may have more taste. A tart lemon custard might

taste good and will also provide needed protein and calories. *(Do not try this if you have a sore mouth or throat.)*

- Serve foods at room temperature.
- Try using bacon, ham, or onion to add flavor to vegetables.
- Stop eating foods that cause an unpleasant taste.

Dry Mouth

Chemotherapy or radiation therapy in the head or neck area, which can reduce the flow of saliva, often cause dry mouth. When this happens, foods are harder to chew and swallow. Dry mouth can also change the way foods taste. The suggestions below may be helpful in dealing with dry mouth. Also try some of the ideas for dealing with a sore mouth or throat, which can make foods easier to swallow.

- Try very sweet or tart foods and beverages such as lemonade; these foods may help your mouth produce more saliva. *(Do not try this if you are also suffering from a tender mouth or sore throat.)*
- Suck on hard candy (preferably sugar-free candy that won't cause tooth decay) or popsicles or chew sugar-free gum, which also can help produce more saliva.
- Use soft and pureed foods, which may be easier to swallow.
- Keep your lips moist with lip salves.
- Eat foods with sauces, gravies, and salad dressings to make them moist and easier to swallow.
- Have a sip of water every few minutes to help you swallow and talk more easily.
- If your dry mouth problem is severe, ask your doctor or dentist about products that coat and protect your mouth and throat.

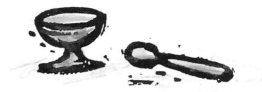

Nausea, with or without vomiting, is a common side effect of surgery, chemotherapy, radiation therapy, and immunotherapy. The disease itself, or other conditions unrelated to your cancer or treatment, may also cause nausea.

Whatever the cause, nausea can keep you from getting enough food and needed nutrients. Here are some ideas that may be helpful:

- Ask your doctor about medicine to help control nausea.
- Try foods such as:
  —Toast and crackers.
  —Yogurt.
  —Sherbet.
  —Pretzels.
  —Angelfood cake.
  —Oatmeal.
  —Skinned chicken (baked or broiled, not fried).
  —Fruits and vegetables that are soft or bland, such as canned peaches.
  —Clear liquids, sipped slowly.
  —Ice chips.
- Avoid foods such as:
  —Fatty, greasy, or fried foods.
  —Very sweet foods such as candy, cookies, or cake.
  —Spicy, hot foods.
  —Foods with strong odors.
- Eat small amounts often and slowly.
- Avoid eating in a room that's stuffy, too warm, or has cooking odors or smells that might disagree with you.
- Drink fewer liquids with meals; drinking liquids can cause a full, bloated feeling.
- Drink or sip liquids throughout the day, *except* at mealtimes. Using a straw may help.
- Drink beverages cool or chilled. Try freezing favorite beverages in ice cube trays.
- Eat foods at room temperature or cooler; hot foods may add to nausea.

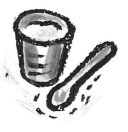

- Don't force yourself to eat favorite foods when you feel nauseated; it may cause a permanent dislike of those foods.
- Rest after meals, because activity may slow digestion. It's best to rest sitting up for about an hour after meals.
- If nausea is a problem in the morning, try eating dry toast or crackers before getting up.
- Wear loose-fitting clothes.
- Avoid eating for 1 to 2 hours before treatment if nausea occurs during radiation therapy or chemotherapy.
- Try to keep track of when your nausea occurs and what causes it (specific foods, events, surroundings). If possible, make appropriate changes in your diet or schedule. Share the information with your doctor or nurse.

Vomiting

Vomiting may follow nausea and may be brought on by treatment, food odors, gas in the stomach or bowel, or motion. In some people, certain surroundings (such as the hospital) may cause vomiting.

If vomiting is severe or lasts for more than a few days, contact your doctor.

Very often, if you can control nausea, you can prevent vomiting. At times though, you may not be able to prevent either nausea or vomiting. You may find some relief by using relaxation exercises or meditation. These usually involve deep rhythmic breathing and quiet concentration and can be done almost anywhere. If vomiting occurs, try these hints to prevent further episodes.

- Ask your doctor about medicine to control nausea.
- Do not drink or eat until you have the vomiting under control.
- Once you have controlled vomiting, try small amounts of clear liquids. Begin with a teaspoonful every 10 minutes, gradually increase

the amount to a tablespoonful every 20 minutes, and finally, try 2 tablespoonfuls every 30 minutes.

■ When you are able to keep down clear liquids, try a full-liquid diet. Continue taking small amounts as often as you can keep them down. If you feel okay on a full-liquid diet, gradually work up to your regular diet. (You can find information about special diets under "Special Diets for Special Needs" on page 27.)

Diarrhea

Diarrhea may have several causes, including chemotherapy, radiation therapy to the abdomen, infection, food sensitivity, and emotional upset.

Long-term or severe diarrhea may cause other problems. During diarrhea food passes quickly through the bowel before the body gets enough vitamins, minerals, and water. This may cause dehydration (when your body doesn't have enough water) and increase the risk of infection. Contact your doctor if the diarrhea is severe or lasts for more than a couple of days. Here are some ideas for coping with diarrhea:

■ Try foods that are high in protein and calories, but low in fiber.
—Yogurt.
—Rice or noodles.
—Applesauce, grape juice.
—Farina or cream of wheat.
—Eggs (cooked until the whites are solid, not fried).
—Ripe bananas.
—Pureed vegetables.
—Canned or cooked fruit without skins.
—Smooth peanut butter.
—White bread.
—Chicken or turkey, skinned.
—Tender or ground beef.
—Fish.
—Cottage cheese, cream cheese.

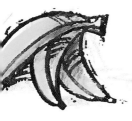

- Elimate foods such as:
  —Greasy, fatty, or fried foods.
  —Raw vegetables and fruits.
  —High-fiber vegetables such as broccoli, corn, beans, cabbage, peas, and cauliflower.
  —Strong spices, such as hot pepper, curry, and Cajun spice mix.
- Eat small amounts of food and liquids throughout the day instead of three large meals.
- Drink plenty of liquids during the day, *except* at mealtimes. Drinking fluids is important because your body may not get enough water when you have diarrhea. Avoid carbonated drinks, such as soda, which can worsen diarrhea.
- Drink liquids that are at room temperature. Avoid very hot or very cold foods.
- Eat plenty of foods and liquids that contain sodium (salt) and potassium. These minerals are often lost during diarrhea. Good liquid choices include bouillon or fat-free broth. Foods high in potassium that don't cause diarrhea include bananas, peach and apricot nectar, and boiled or mashed potatoes.
- After sudden, short-term attacks of diarrhea (acute diarrhea), try a clear-liquid diet during the first 12 to 14 hours. This lets the bowel rest while replacing the important body fluids lost during diarrhea. (Guidelines for a clear-liquid diet appear on pages 28-29.)
- Limit foods and beverages that contain caffeine, such as coffee, strong tea, some sodas, and chocolate.
- Be careful when using milk and milk products, because diarrhea may be caused by lactose intolerance when you can't digest the lactose in milk. If you think you have this problem, see "Low-Lactose Diet" on page 38. Also, ask your doctor or dietitian for advice.

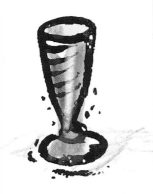

Constipation

Some anticancer drugs and other drugs, such as pain medicines, may cause constipation. This problem also may occur if your diet lacks enough fluid or bulk or if you have been bedridden.

Here are some suggestions to prevent and treat constipation:

- Drink plenty of liquids, *except* at mealtime. This will help to keep stools soft.
- Take a hot drink about one-half hour before your usual time for a bowel movement.
- Eat high-fiber foods such as whole grains, and raw fresh vegetables and fruits such as cauliflower, potatoes with skin, peas, bananas, pears, oranges, and berries.
- Get some exercise, such as walking, every day. Talk to your doctor or a physical therapist about the amount and type of exercise that is right for you.
- Add wheat bran to foods such as casseroles and homemade breads.

If none of these suggestions works, ask your doctor about medicine to ease constipation. *Be sure to check with your doctor before taking any laxatives or stool softeners.*

Weight Gain

Sometimes patients gain excess weight during treatment without eating extra calories. For example, certain anticancer drugs (such as prednisone) can cause the body to hold on to fluid and, thus, to gain weight. The extra weight is in the form of water and does not mean you are eating too much.

It is important not to go on a diet if you notice weight gain. Instead, tell your doctor so you can find out what may be causing this change. If anticancer drugs cause weight gain, the doctor may recommend limiting the salt you eat because salt causes your body to hold on to water. Drugs called diuretics also may be prescribed to get rid of extra fluid.

Tooth Decay

Cancer and cancer treatment can cause tooth decay and other problems for your teeth and gums. Changes in eating habits also may add to the problem. If you eat often or eat a lot of sweets, you may need to brush your teeth more often. Brushing after each meal or snack is a good idea.

Here are some ideas for preventing dental problems:

- Be sure to see your dentist regularly. Patients who are receiving treatment that affects the mouth (e.g., radiation to the head and neck) may need to see the dentist more often than usual.

- Use a soft toothbrush. If your gums are very sensitive, clean your teeth with cotton swabs or mouthswabs made especially for teeth cleaning.

- Rinse your mouth with warm water when your gums and mouth are sore.

- If you are not having trouble with poor appetite or weight loss, limit the amount of sugar in your diet.

- Avoid eating foods that stick to the teeth such as caramels or chewy candy bars.

Lactose Intolerance

Lactose intolerance means that your body can't digest or absorb the milk sugar called lactose. Milk, other dairy products, and foods to which milk has been added contain lactose.

Lactose intolerance may occur after treatment with some antibiotics or with radiation to the stomach or any treatment that affects the digestive tract. The part of your intestines that breaks down lactose may not work properly during treatment. For some people the symptoms (gas, cramping, diarrhea) disappear a few weeks or months after the treatments end or when the intestine heals. For others a permanent change in eating habits may be needed.

If you have this problem, your doctor may advise you to follow a diet that is low in foods that contain lactose. (See "Low-Lactose Diet" on page 39.) If milk had been a main source of protein in your diet, it will be important to get enough protein from other foods.

Products such as soybean formulas and aged cheeses are good sources of protein and other nutrients. The recipes beginning on page 53 give you ideas for preparing low-lactose dishes.

**Improving
Your Nutrition**

There are many ways to improve your nutrition in order to lessen the side effects of your treatment. Table 1 provides a list of healthy snacks. Tables 2 and 3 on the following pages offer ideas for increasing protein and calories in your diet. There are also hints for saving time and energy in preparing meals.

When side effects of treatment occur, they usually go away after treatment ends. Long-term treatment, however, may mean long-term changes to your diet to help you continue to handle side effects and keep up your strength.

The ideas and suggestions listed here have worked for other cancer patients during their treatment. Each person is different, though, and you will have to find out what works best for you.

**Saving Time
and Energy**

Your body needs both rest and nourishment during and after treatment for cancer. If you are usually the cook, here are some suggestions for saving time and energy in preparing meals.

- Let someone else do the cooking when possible.

- If you know that your recovery time from treatment or surgery is going to be longer than 1 or 2 days, prepare a helper list. Decide who can help you shop, cook, set the table, and clean up. Write it down, discuss it, and post it where it can easily be seen. If children help, plan a small reward for them.

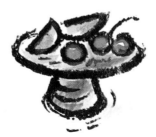

TABLE 1. HEALTHY SNACKS

Have these on hand for quick and easy nibbles:

Applesauce
Bread products, including
  muffins and crackers
Buttered popcorn
Cake and cookies made with
  whole grains, fruits, nuts,
  wheat germ, or granola
Cereal
Cheese, hard or semisoft
Cheesecake
Chocolate milk
Cottage cheese
Cream cheese and other
  soft cheese
Cream soups
Dips made with cheese, beans,
  or sour cream

Dried fruits such as raisins,
  prunes, or apricots
Fruits (fresh or canned)
Gelatin salads and desserts
Granola
Hard-boiled and deviled eggs
Ice cream, frozen yogurt, popsicles
Juices
Nuts
Peanut butter
Pizza
Puddings and custards
Quesadillas
Sandwiches
Vegetables (raw or cooked)
Whole-milk milkshakes/instant
  breakfast
Yogurt, regular or frozen

- Write out menus, choosing things that you or your family can put together easily. Casseroles, TV dinners, hot dogs, hamburgers, and meals that you have prepared and frozen ahead are all good ideas. Cook larger batches to be frozen so you will have them for future use. Add instructions so that other people can help you.

- Use shopping lists. Keep them handy so that they can be used as guides either by you or other people.

- When making casseroles for freezing, only partially cook rice and macaroni products. They will cook further in the reheating process. Add ½ cup liquid to refrigerated or frozen casseroles when reheating because they can get dry during refrigeration. Remember that frozen casseroles take a long time to heat completely—at least 45 minutes in deep dishes in the oven.

- Don't be shy about accepting gifts of food and offers of help from family and friends. Let them know what you like and offer your recipes. If people bring food you can't use right away, freeze it. That homecooked meal can break the monotony of quickie suppers. It can also save time when you're on a tight schedule. Date the food when you put it in the refrigerator or freezer.

- Have as few dishes, pots, and pans to wash as possible. Cook in dishes and pans that can also make attractive servers. Use paper napkins and disposable dishes, especially for dessert. Paper cups are fine for kids and for medicines. Disposable pans are a great timesaver—foil containers from frozen foods make good disposable pans. Soak dirty dishes to cut down washing time.

- When you are preparing soft dishes, choose foods that the whole family can eat such as omelets, scrambled eggs, macaroni and cheese, meatloaf, tuna salad sandwiches, or tuna casseroles. Set aside enough food to be pureed in the blender or food processor for yourself.

- Use mixes, frozen ready-to-eat main dishes, and takeout foods whenever possible. The less time spent cooking and cleaning up, the more time for relaxation and the family.

- If someone is cooking for you, share this booklet with them for ideas for food selection and preparation. They will also get a better sense of your special needs.

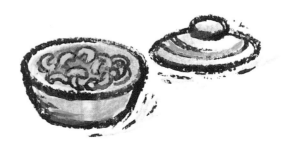

TABLE 2. HOW TO INCREASE PROTEIN

Hard or Semisoft Cheese
(e.g., cheddar, Jack, brick)

- Melt on sandwiches, bread, muffins, tortillas, hamburgers, hot dogs, other meats or fish, vegetables, eggs, and desserts such as stewed fruit or pies.
- Grate and add to soups, sauces, casseroles, vegetable dishes, mashed potatoes, rice, noodles, or meatloaf.

Cottage Cheese/ Ricotta Cheese

- Mix with or use to stuff fruits and vegetables.
- Add to casseroles, spaghetti, noodles, and egg dishes such as omelets, scrambled eggs, and souffles.
- Use in gelatin, pudding-type desserts, cheesecake, and pancake batter.
- Use to stuff crepes and pasta shells or manicotti.

Milk

- Use milk in beverages and in cooking when possible.
- Use in preparing foods such as hot cereal, soups, cocoa, or pudding.
- Add cream sauces to vegetable and other dishes.
- Add a tablespoon of nonfat dry powdered milk to each cup of regular milk, cream soups, and mashed potatoes.

Powdered Milk

- Add to regular milk and milk drinks such as pasteurized eggnog and milkshakes.
- Use in casseroles, meatloaf, breads, muffins, sauces, cream soups, puddings and custards, and milk-based desserts.

Commercial Products

- See the section on "Commercial Products to Improve Nutrition" on page 42 and table 4, "Nutritional Products Commonly Available in Supermarkets and Drugstores," also on page 42.
- Use instant breakfast powder in milk drinks and desserts.
- Mix with ice cream, milk, and fruit or flavorings for a high-protein milkshake.

Ice Cream, Yogurt, and Frozen Yogurt

- Add to carbonated beverages such as gingerale; add to milk drinks such as milkshakes.
- Add to cereals, fruits, gelatin desserts, and pies; blend or whip with soft or cooked fruits.
- Sandwich ice cream or frozen yogurt between enriched cake slices, cookies, or graham crackers.

TABLE 2. Continued

Eggs and Egg Yolks	■ Add chopped, hard-cooked eggs to salads and dressings, vegetables, casseroles, and creamed meats. ■ Beat eggs into mashed potatoes, vegetable purees, and sauces. Add extra yolks to quiches, scrambled eggs, custards, puddings, pancake and french toast batter, and milkshakes. ■ Make a rich custard with egg yolks, high-protein milk, and sugar. ■ Add extra hard-cooked yolks to deviled egg filling and sandwich spreads.
Nuts, Seeds, and Wheat Germ	■ Add to casseroles, breads, muffins, pancakes, cookies, and waffles. ■ Sprinkle on fruit, cereal, ice cream, yogurt, vegetables, salads, and toast as a crunchy topping; use in place of bread crumbs. ■ Blend with parsley or spinach, herbs, and cream for a noodle, pasta, or vegetable sauce. ■ Roll banana in chopped nuts.
Peanut Butter	■ Spread on sandwiches, toast, muffins, crackers, waffles, pancakes, and fruit slices. ■ Use as a dip for raw vegetables such as carrots, cauliflower, and celery. ■ Blend with milk drinks and beverages. ■ Swirl through soft ice cream and yogurt.
Meat and Fish	■ Add chopped cooked meat or fish to vegetables, salads, casseroles, soups, sauces, and biscuit dough. ■ Use in omelets, souffles, quiches, sandwich fillings, and chicken and turkey stuffings. ■ Wrap in piecrust or biscuit dough as turnovers. ■ Add to stuffed baked potatoes. ■ Eat calves or chicken liver or heart, which are especially good sources of protein, vitamins, and minerals.
Beans	■ Cook and use dried peas and beans and bean curd (tofu) in soups or add to casseroles, pastas, and grain dishes that also contain cheese or meat. Mash with cheese and milk.

TABLE 3. HOW TO INCREASE CALORIES

Butter and Margarine
- Add to soups, mashed and baked potatoes, hot cereals, grits, rice, noodles, and cooked vegetables.
- Stir into cream soups, sauces, and gravies.
- Combine with herbs and seasonings and spread on cooked meats, hamburgers, and fish and egg dishes.
- Use melted butter or margarine as a dip for raw vegetables and seafoods such as shrimp, scallops, crab, and lobster.

Whipped Cream
- Use sweetened on hot chocolate, desserts, gelatin, puddings, fruits, pancakes, and waffles.
- Fold unsweetened into mashed potatoes or vegetable purees.

Table Cream
- Use in cream soups, sauces, egg dishes, batters, puddings, and custards.
- Put on hot or cold cereal.
- Mix with pasta, rice, and mashed potatoes.
- Pour on chicken and fish while baking.
- Use as a binder in hamburgers, meatloaf, and croquettes.
- Add to milk in recipes.
- Make hot chocolate with cream and add marshmallows.

Cream Cheese
- Spread on breads, muffins, fruit slices, and crackers.
- Add to vegetables.
- Roll into balls and coat with chopped nuts, wheat germ, or granola.

Sour Cream
- Add to cream soups, baked potatoes, macaroni and cheese, vegetables, sauces, salad dressings, stews, baked meat, and fish.
- Use as a topping for cakes, fruit, gelatin desserts, breads, and muffins.
- Use as a dip for fresh fruits and vegetables.
- For a good dessert, scoop it on fresh fruit, add brown sugar, and let it sit in the refrigerator for a while.

TABLE 3. Continued

Salad Dressings and Mayonnaise	■ Spread on sandwiches and crackers. ■ Combine with meat, fish, and egg or vegetable salads. ■ Use as a binder in croquettes. ■ Use in sauces and gelatin dishes.
Honey, Jam, and Sugar	■ Add to bread, cereal, milk drinks, and fruit and yogurt desserts. ■ Use as a glaze for meats such as chicken.
Granola	■ Use in cookie, muffin, and bread batters. ■ Sprinkle on vegetables, yogurt, ice cream, pudding, custard, and fruit. ■ Layer with fruits and bake. ■ Mix with dry fruits and nuts for a snack. ■ Substitute for bread or rice in pudding recipes.
Dried Fruits	■ Cook and serve for breakfast or as a dessert or snack. ■ Add to muffins, cookies, breads, cakes, rice and grain dishes, cereals, puddings, and stuffings. ■ Bake in pies and turnovers. ■ Combine with cooked vegetables such as carrots, sweet potatoes, yams, and acorn and butternut squash. ■ Combine with nuts or granola for snacks.
Food Preparation	■ Bread meats and vegetables. ■ Saute and fry foods when possible, because these cooking methods add more calories than baking or broiling. ■ Add sauces or gravies.

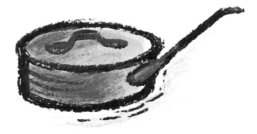

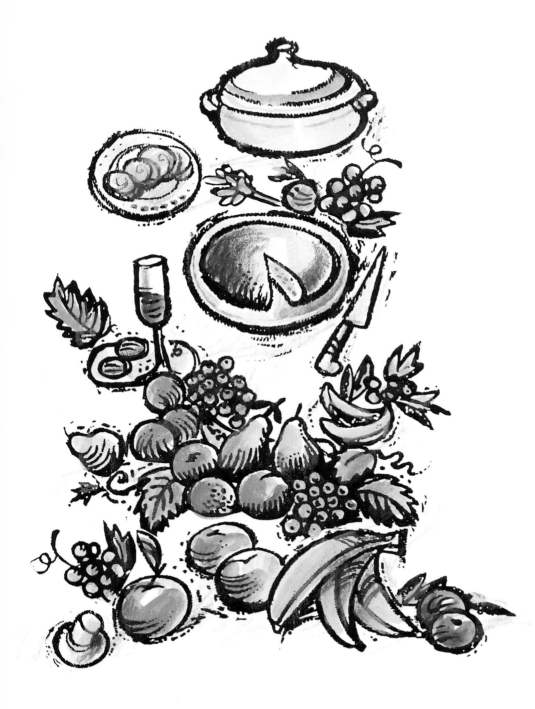

Special Diets for Special Needs

When you can't eat enough, your doctor may prescribe a special diet. Your doctor also may suggest a commercial product to help nutrition. In the following sections, you will find guidelines for several special diets used during cancer treatment. You will also learn about products that can boost nutrition and where you can buy them. *Remember that special diets and products to improve nutrition should be used only as recommended by your doctor or registered dietitian.*

Special diets are an important tool for correcting nutritional problems that occur during cancer treatment. Patients may follow some of these diets only for a few days; they may not provide enough nutrients for the long term. Only your doctor, nurse, or registered dietitian should decide whether you need a special diet and for how long. If you are already following a special diet for another health problem, you and your doctor and registered dietitian should work together to develop your new plan.

Guidelines for common special diets appear in this section, including:

- Clear-liquid diet.
- Full-liquid diet.
- Soft diet.
- Low-residue diet.
- Low-lactose diet.

For each diet, you will find a brief explanation of when doctors use the diet, the major foods it includes, and a suggested meal pattern. In addition, the section contains a tear-out diet sheet that you can display in the kitchen or keep for handy reference.

This information will help you follow the diet recommended by your doctor. If you think you need a special diet, talk with your doctor or dietitian.

CLEAR-LIQUID DIET

Type of Food	Allowed Items	Excluded Items
Beverages	Water, carbonated beverages; cereal beverages; coffee, tea;* fruit-flavored drinks; strained lemonade, limeade, and fruit punches	Milk, milk drinks, all others**
Breads Cereals Flours	None	All
Cheeses	None	All
Desserts	Plain gelatin desserts, fruit ices without milk or pieces of fruit, popsicles	All others
Eggs	None	All
Fats	None	All
Fruits Fruit Juices	Apple, cranberry, grape juice; strained citrus juices if tolerated	All others

Clear-Liquid Diet

Clear-liquid diets are useful if the body can't handle the softest foods or heavy or thick liquids. Patients usually follow this type of diet after surgery or before stomach or bowel surgery. Patients with severe nausea and vomiting may also have this diet. A clear-liquid diet often lasts 1 to 2 days or until you can drink or eat other beverages and foods. It cannot meet the suggested daily servings on pages 4 and 5 (except for fruit juices), but it helps ensure that your body doesn't lose too much fluid as you recover and become ready for a regular diet.

CLEAR-LIQUID DIET *Continued*

Type of Food	Allowed Items	Excluded Items
Meat **Poultry** **Fish** **Legumes**	None	All
Milk **Milk Products**	None	All
Potatoes **Rice** **Pasta**	None	All
Soup	Bouillon, clear fat-free broths, consomme	All others
Sweets	Honey, jelly, syrups, plain sugar candy in small amounts	All others
Vegetables	Strained vegetable broth	All others
Miscellaneous	Salt	All others

Your doctor may recommend decaffeinated coffee or tea.
**Check with your doctor about alcohol. Alcohol cannot be used safely with some medicines.*

CLEAR-LIQUID DIET *Suggested Meal Pattern*

Breakfast

1 cup juice
1 cup clear broth
½ cup gelatin dessert
Coffee or tea* with sugar

A.M. Snack

1 cup fruit juice or soft drink
½ cup gelatin dessert

Lunch

1 cup juice
1 cup clear broth
½ cup gelatin dessert
Coffee or tea* with sugar

P.M. Snack

1 cup fruit juice or soft
   drink
½ cup gelatin dessert

Dinner

1 cup juice
1 cup clear broth
½ cup gelatin dessert
Coffee or tea* with sugar

Evening Snack

1 cup fruit juice or soft
   drink
½ cup gelatin dessert

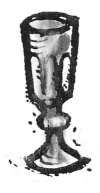

FULL-LIQUID DIET

Type of Food	Allowed Items	Excluded Items
Beverages	Cereal beverages; coffee, tea;* fruit drinks; strained lemonade, limeade, or fruit punches; water	None**
Breads Cereals Flours	Refined or strained cooked cereal	Breads and cereals in solid form
Cheeses	Cheese soup	All others
Desserts	Plain gelatin desserts, junket, soft or baked custards, sherbets, plain cornstarch pudding, fresh or frozen yogurt, ice milk, smooth ice cream	All others, particularly those with fruits or seeds
Eggs	Pasteurized eggnog	All others
Fats	Butter, cream, oils, margarine	All others
Fruits Fruit Juices	All juices and nectars, thin fruit purees	All others
Meat Poultry Fish Legumes	Small amounts of strained meat in broth or gelatin	All others

Full-Liquid Diet

You may follow a full-liquid diet when your body can digest all liquids but can't handle solid food yet. Your doctor may recommend this diet after surgery or when you can't chew and swallow food. All liquids served at room or body temperature are part of this diet. This diet can include most of the recommended food groups on pages 4 and 5, except meat. Extra milk has been included to ensure adequate protein. When planned properly, this diet can be used for long periods. In these instances, your doctor may prescribe a commercial supplement and/or certain vitamins. However, you should only take these if your doctor recommends them.

If you must follow a full-liquid diet over a long period, you can increase the protein and calorie content of the diet by:

FULL-LIQUID DIET *Continued*

Type of Food	Allowed Items	Excluded Items
Milk **Milk Products**	Chocolate, buttermilk, skim, and whole milk; ice milk; milkshakes; plain yogurt	All others, yogurt with pieces of fruit
Potatoes **Rice** **Pasta**	Potatoes pureed in soup	All others
Soups	Bouillon, broth, clear cream soups, any strained or blenderized soup	All others
Sweets	Honey, jelly, syrups in small amounts	All others
Vegetables	Tomato puree for cream soups; tomato, vegetable juices	All others
Miscellaneous	Flavoring extracts, salt	All others

*Your doctor may recommend decaffeinated coffee or tea.

**Check with your doctor before drinking alcohol. Alcohol cannot be used safely with some medicines.

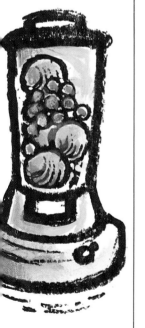

FULL-LIQUID DIET *Suggested Meal Pattern*

Breakfast

1 cup fruit juice
1 cup strained cereal
1 cup milk
Coffee or tea* with sugar

A.M. Snack

1 cup fruit juice

Lunch

1 cup strained soup (made with vegetable puree)
1 cup strained cereal
½ cup allowed dessert
1 cup fruit juice
1 cup milk or yogurt
Coffee or tea* with sugar

P.M. Snack

1 cup milk or eggnog

Dinner

1 cup strained cream soup (with a small amount of strained meat)
1 cup milk
1 cup strained cereal
½ cup allowed dessert
1 cup vegetable juice
Coffee or tea* with sugar

Evening Snack

1 cup milk or yogurt

- Adding nonfat dry milk to beverages and soups.
- Adding strained meats (such as those in baby food) to broths.

You can increase the calories of a full-liquid diet by:

- Adding butter to hot cereal and soups.
- Including sugar or syrup (glucose) in beverages.
- Using smooth ice cream in desserts and beverages.
- Using prepared breakfast mixes in milk or milkshakes.

You will find other helpful ideas in table 2 "How To Increase Protein" and table 3 "How To Increase Calories" in the section "Choosing Foods for Better Nutrition."

Soft Diet

A soft diet is useful when your body is ready for more than liquids but still unable to handle a regular solid diet. Soft food is easier to eat than regular food when the mouth, throat, esophagus, and/or stomach are sore. This can occur after radiation therapy to these parts of the body or during chemotherapy. A soft diet can be used for long periods because it contains all needed nutrients. The diet consists of bland, lower fat foods that you soften by cooking, mashing, pureeing, or blending. Avoid fried or greasy foods and foods that may cause gas.

SOFT DIET

Type of Food	Allowed Items	Excluded Items
Beverages	All	None*
Breads	French, vienna, italian, seedless rye, white, refined whole-wheat, cornbread, or any except whole-grain; if tolerated, muffins, french toast, crackers, biscuits, rolls, pancakes, waffles	Brown, cracked wheat, pumpernickel, raisin, rye with seeds, buckwheat; whole-grain crackers; rolls with coconut, raisins, nuts, or whole grains; tortillas
Cereals	Refined, cooked, or ready-to-eat	Whole-grain or bran
Flours	All except those excluded	Whole-grain, bran, or wheat
Cheeses	All except those excluded	Sharp or strongly flavored cheeses; those containing whole seeds and spices
Desserts	Ice milk, ice cream, sherbet, ices, custards, gelatins, or others with allowed fruits	Desserts made with excluded fruits, nuts, coconut
Eggs	All except those excluded	Raw, fried
Fats	Butter, cream, cream substitutes, vegetable shortening and oils, margarine, mayonnaise, sour cream, commercial french dressing	Other salad dressings; salt pork; fried foods
Fruits **Fruit Juices**	All juices and nectars; avocado, banana, canned or cooked apples, apricots, cherries, grapefruit and orange sections without membrane, peaches, pears, seedless grapes	All raw fruit except avocado and banana; all dried fruit; berries, crabapples, coconut, figs, grapes, melons, pineapples, plums, rhubarb
Meat	Tender beef, lamb, veal, or liver that is baked, broiled, creamed, roasted, or stewed; roasted or stewed pork	Fried, salted, and smoked meats; chitterlings, corned beef, sausage, cold cuts
Poultry	Chicken, cornish game hen, turkey, chicken livers	Duck, goose; fried poultry

SOFT DIET *Continued*

Type of Food	Allowed Items	Excluded Items
Fish	Cooked, fresh, or frozen fish without bones; tuna, salmon	Fried fish, shellfish, anchovies, caviar, herring, sardines, snails, skate
Legumes **Nuts**	Creamy peanut butter	All other legumes, nuts, and seed kernels
Milk **Milk Products**	All	None
Potatoes **Rice** **Pasta**	Baked, boiled, creamed, scalloped, mashed, au gratin; mashed sweet potatoes; dumplings; noodles; brown or white rice; spaghetti	French fries, hashbrowns, potato salad, whole sweet potatoes or yams; bread stuffing; fritters; chow mein noodles; wild rice; barley
Soups	Bouillon, broth, consomme, strained cream and vegetable	Bean, split pea, onion; bisques; gumbos; unstrained chowders
Sweets	Apple butter, butterscotch candy, caramels, chocolate, fondant, plain fudge, lollipops, marshmallows, mints, honey, jelly, syrups, sugars in small amounts	Candied fruits, nut brittle, jams, preserves, marmalade, marzipan, fruit sauces with prohibited fruits
Vegetables	Canned or cooked asparagus, beans, carrots, beets, eggplant, mushrooms, parsley, pumpkin, spinach, squash, tomatoes, tomato juice, vegetable juice cocktail, raw lettuce if tolerated	All raw vegetables except lettuce; all canned or cooked vegetables not specifically listed as allowed
Miscellaneous	Aspic, catsup, gelatin, gravy, pretzels, soy sauce, vinegar; brown, cheese, cream, tomato, and white sauces; all finely chopped or ground leaf herbs and spices	Garlic, horseradish, olives, pickles, popcorn, potato chips, relishes, chili, a-la-king, creole, barbecue, cocktail, sweet-and-sour, Newburg, Worcestershire sauces, whole and seed herbs and spices

Check with your doctor before drinking alcohol. Alcohol cannot be used safely with some medicines.

SOFT DIET *Suggested Meal Pattern*

Breakfast

½ cup fruit or juice
½ to 1 cup cereal
2 eggs, scrambled
1 slice toast
1 tsp. butter or margarine
Jelly
1 cup milk
Sugar and cream

Lunch

½ cup fruit juice
2 oz. meat, fish, or poultry
½ cup vegetable
2 slices bread
1 tsp. butter or margarine
1 serving fruit or allowed dessert
1 cup milk

Dinner

4 oz. meat, fish, or poultry
1 cup potato
½ cup vegetable
1 slice bread or roll
1 tsp. butter or margarine
1 serving fruit or allowed dessert
1 c. milk, milkshake, or eggnog

Snack

½ cup fruit or allowed dessert

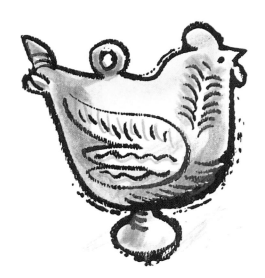

Low-Residue Diet

Your doctor may recommend a low-residue diet after radiation therapy to the bowel. It also is helpful when excess fiber or milk products irritate the bowel and cause diarrhea and/or cramping.

Your registered dietitian may gradually increase fiber and milk products in this diet according to how well you handle them.

LOW-RESIDUE DIET

Type of Food	Allowed Items	Excluded Items
Beverages	Fruit flavored drinks, milk drinks (2 cups milk or milk products allowed per day), carbonated beverages, coffee, tea;* all others no limitation	None**
Breads	French, vienna, italian, refined whole-wheat, white, and rye breads without seeds; crackers; biscuits; french toast; plain hard crust, zwieback rolls	Breads, crackers, rolls, or cereals containing whole-grain or graham flour, bran, seeds, nuts, or raisins; cornbread
Cereals	All refined, cooked, or dry cereals; oatmeal	All cereals made from prohibited flours or other foods
Flours	All except those excluded	Bran, graham, whole-wheat, or whole-grain flours
Cheeses	Cottage, cream, American, swiss, muenster, or other mild cheese; 1 oz. may be substituted for 1 cup milk	All others
Desserts	Custards, gelatin puddings, plain cookies and cakes, sherbets, pastry without nuts	All desserts containing seeds, nuts, coconut, or raisins; tough-skinned fruits
Eggs	All except fried	Fried eggs
Fats	Crisp bacon, butter, oils, cream, dry cream substitutes, margarine, mayonnaise, shortenings, smooth salad dressings, sour cream	Salad dressing made with excluded foods; tartar sauce
Fruits **Fruit Juices**	All juices and nectars; canned or cooked fruit; peeled fruit without seeds; apples, applesauce, apricots, avocados, bananas, cherries, grapefruit, oranges, tangerines, fruit cocktail, grapes, melons, cantaloupe, honeydew, peaches, pears, pineapple, plums (2 servings allowed per day)	All other fresh fruits, dried fruits, berries, figs, grapes with seeds

LOW-RESIDUE DIET *Continued*

Type of Food	Allowed Items	Excluded Items
Meat **Poultry**	Tender beef, ham, lamb, liver, poultry, or veal that is baked, broiled, or stewed	Fried meats and poultry, smoked or cured meats, cold cuts, corned beef, frankfurters, pastrami, sausage
Fish	Fresh or frozen fish without bones, canned tuna or salmon, cooked shellfish	All fried or smoked fish, sardines, herring
Legumes **Nuts**	None	All dried legumes, lima beans, peas, nuts
Milk **Milk Products**	Buttermilk, chocolate, skim, and whole milk; yogurt (2 cups, including that used in cooking, allowed per day)	Yogurt containing fruits
Potatoes **Rice** **Pasta**	Boiled, creamed, mashed, and scalloped potatoes (without skin); macaroni, noodles, white rice, spaghetti (1 serving potato allowed per day; all others, no limitation)	Potato skin, potato cakes, french fries, hashbrowns, potato salad, sweet potato, brown and wild rice, barley, hominy
Soups	Cream and broth-based soups made with allowed foods	All others
Sweets	Honey, jelly, syrup, candy	Jams, preserves, candies with fruits, coconut, raisins, nuts, candied fruits
Vegetables	Canned or cooked asparagus, beans, beets, carrots, mushrooms, peas, pumpkin, squash, spinach, tomatoes, turnip greens, tomato juice, raw lettuce if tolerated (no limitation on juices; 1 serving whole vegetables allowed per day)	All raw vegetables except lettuce; canned or cooked vegetables not specifically allowed
Miscellaneous	Ground or finely chopped herbs and spices, salt, flavoring extracts, catsup, chocolate, mild gravy, white sauce, soy sauce, vinegar	All other spices and condiments, olives, pickles, potato chips, popcorn

*Your doctor may recommend decaffeinated coffee or tea.
**Check with your doctor before drinking alcohol. Alcohol cannot be used safely with some medicines.

LOW-RESIDUE *Suggested Meal Pattern*

Breakfast

½ cup strained fruit juice*
1 serving allowed cereal
1 egg
2 strips crisp bacon
1 slice toast
1 tsp. butter or margarine
Jelly
1 cup milk**
Sugar

Lunch

½ cup soup
2 oz. meat, poultry, or fish
½ cup allowed vegetable
2 slices bread or roll
2 tsp. butter or margarine
1 serving allowed dessert

Dinner

5 oz. lean meat, poultry, or fish
2 slices bread or roll
1 cup milk**
3 tsp. butter or margarine
1 baked potato, without skin
1 serving allowed dessert
½ cup vegetable juice

Snack

½ cup fruit juice*
3 plain cookies

*2 servings of fruit/juices allowed per day.
**2 servings of milk products allowed per day.

Low-Lactose Diet

All milk products contain lactose (or milk sugar). The doctor may recommend a low-lactose diet after radiation therapy to the intestines, which often makes lactose hard to digest for a time. Fermented milk products, such as buttermilk, sour cream, and yogurt, are often easier to handle than whole milk. Lactose is often a filler in many products such as instant coffee and some medicines. Read labels on commercial foods carefully.

Lactose tolerance varies from person to person. Ask your doctor or registered dietitian about choosing allowed foods.

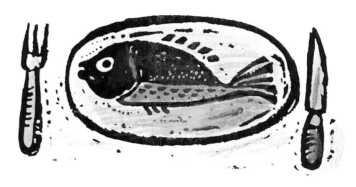

LOW-LACTOSE DIET

Type of Food	Allowed Items	Excluded Items
Beverages	Water, lactose-free carbonated beverages, fruit-flavored drinks, fruit punches, lemonade, limeade, nondairy product drinks, coffee and tea*	Artificial fruit drinks containing lactose, all beverages made with milk and milk products with the exception of buttermilk or yogurt**
Bread	All	None
Cereals	Any cooked or dry cereal not containing lactose	Instant hot cereals, high-protein cereals, all cereals with added milk or lactose
Flours	All	None
Cheeses	Fermented cheeses (cheddar and any cheese aged with bacteria)	All others
Desserts	Fruit ices; gelatins; angelfood cake; desserts made with nondairy products, buttermilk, or sour cream	Ice cream, puddings, and other desserts containing milk or milk products
Eggs	All except eggs prepared with milk or milk products	Creamed, scrambled, omelets, or other eggs prepared with milk
Fats	Margarine not containing milk solids, vegetable oils, mayonnaise, shortening	All others: cream, half-and-half, table and whipping cream, butter
Fruits **Fruit Juices**	All fresh, canned, or frozen fruit juices; fruits not processed with lactose	Any canned or frozen fruits and fruit juices processed with lactose
Meat **Poultry** **Fish** **Legumes** **Nuts**	Any except those specifically excluded	Creamed or breaded fish, poultry, meat; coldcuts, hot dogs, liver, sausage, or other processed meats containing milk or lactose; gravies made with milk
Milk **Milk Products**	Fermented milk products such as acidophilus milk, buttermilk, yogurt, and sour cream	All milk, milk products except fermented milk products

LOW-LACTOSE DIET *Continued*

Type of Food	Allowed Items	Excluded Items
Potatoes **Rice** **Pasta**	White or sweet potatoes, macaroni, noodles, spaghetti or other pasta, rice	Any prepared with milk such as creamed or scalloped, commercial potato products containing dried milk
Soups	Broth-based soups	Cream soups, chowders, commercially prepared soups that contain milk or milk products
Sweets	Honey, jams, preserves, syrups, molasses	Candy containing lactose, milk, or cocoa; butterscotch candies; caramels; chocolates. Read all labels carefully
Vegetables	All vegetables except those prepared with milk	Any prepared with milk such as creamed or scalloped or any processed vegetables containing lactose
Miscellaneous	Catsup, chili sauce, horseradish, olives, pickles, vinegar, gravies prepared without milk, mustard, all herbs and spices, peanut butter, unbuttered popcorn	Chocolate, cocoa, milk gravies, cream sauces, chewing gum, instant coffee, powdered soft drinks, artificial juices containing milk or lactose

*Your doctor may recommend decaffeinated coffee or tea.
**Check with your doctor before drinking alcohol. Alcohol cannot be used safely with some medicines.

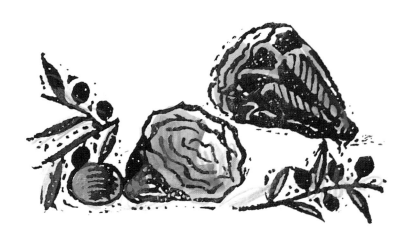

LOW-LACTOSE DIET *Suggested Meal Pattern*

Breakfast

½ cup fruit juice
1 serving cereal
1 egg
2 strips bacon
1 slice toast
1 tsp. margarine*
Jelly
1 cup acidophilus or
  low-lactose milk
Sugar
Salt and pepper

Lunch

½ cup juice and/or broth-
  based soup
3 oz. meat or substitute
½ cup vegetable and/or salad
2 slices bread or roll
2 tsp. margarine*
1 serving fruit or dessert
Salt and pepper
Beverage

Dinner

3 oz. meat or substitute
½ cup potato
½ cup vegetable and/or
  salad
1 slice bread or roll
1 tsp. margarine*
1 serving fruit or dessert
1 cup acidophilus or low-
  lactose milk
Salt and pepper

Snack

½ cup juice

Should not contain milk solids

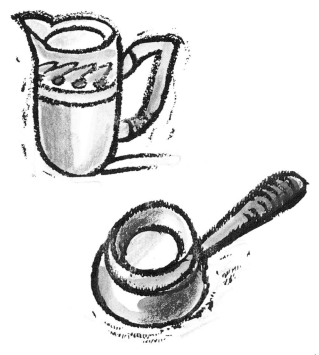

Commercial Products to Improve Nutrition

If you cannot get enough calories and protein from your diet, commercial nutrition supplements, such as formulas and instant breakfast powders, may be helpful. There are also products that can be added to any food or beverage to boost calorie content. These supplements are high in protein and calories and have extra vitamins and minerals. They come in liquid, pudding, and powder forms.

These products need no refrigeration until you open them. Thus, you can carry nutrition supplements with you and take them whenever you feel hungry or thristy. They are good chilled as between-meal and bedtime snacks. You may want to take a can or two with you when you go for treatments or other times when long waits may tire you.

Many supermarkets and drugstores carry these products. Table 4 lists the types of supplements and their calorie and protein contents. (Brand names appear as examples in footnotes. Mention in this booklet does not imply product endorsement, however.)

TABLE 4. **Nutritional Products Commonly Available in Supermarkets and Drugstores**

Type of Product	Serving Size	Calories per Serving	Protein (gms) per Serving
Liquid[1]	8 oz.	180-270	9-14
Liquid, fortified[2]	8 oz.	290-360	14-17
Powder[3]	8-9 oz.	170-280	9-15
Pudding[4]	5 oz.	240	7

[1]*Examples: Sustacal, Isocal, Ensure, Meritene, Sego*
[2]*Examples: Sustacal HC, Ensure Plus, Forta Shake*
[3]*Examples: Instant Breakfast, Meritene, Resource*
[4]*Examples: Forta, Sustacal*

RESOURCES FOR PATIENTS AND FAMILIES

General information about cancer is widely available. Some of the resources and publications listed below might be helpful to you. You may also wish to see what the local library has to offer and contact support groups in your community. You don't have to be an active member of these groups to use their services.

Cancer Information Service (CIS)

The NCI-supported CIS is a nationwide telephone service that responds to inquiries from cancer patients and their families, health care professionals, and the public. Information specialists can provide information and publications on all aspects of cancer. They also may know about cancer support groups and cancer services in your area.

By dialing 1-800-4-CANCER, you will be connected to the CIS office serving your area. Spanish-speaking staff members are available.

Physician Data Query

People who have cancer, those who care about them, and doctors need up-to-date and accurate information about cancer treatment. To help these people, NCI has developed a computer system called Physician Data Query (PDQ). This computer system gives quick and easy access to:

- Cancer treatment information for both patients and doctors.
- Information about research studies, called clinical trials, that test new and promising cancer treatments and are open to patients.
- Names of organizations and doctors who care for people with cancer.

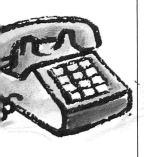

To use PDQ, doctors may use an office computer or the services of a medical library. By calling 1-800-4-CANCER, doctors and patients can get PDQ information as well as learn how to use this system.

Clinical Trials

Clinical trials are carefully designed research studies to test new and promising cancer treatments. Patients who take part in these trials may be the first to benefit from new or improved treatment metods. They also can make an important contribution to medical care because the results of the studies may help many people. Patients participate in clinical trials only if they choose to, and they are free to leave the trial at any time. Further information about these research studies is provided in the booklet *What Are Clinical Trials All About?* To obtain a free copy of this booklet, contact the CIS at 1-800-4-CANCER.

Publications

You also may want to read some other NCI booklets and factsheets that discuss various aspects of cancer, cancer treatment, and patient concerns. The following booklets may be especially helpful:

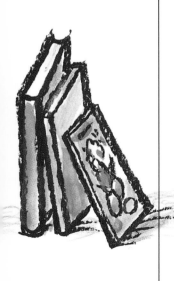

- *What You Need to Know About...*This is a series of booklets about different types of cancer. Specify a primary cancer site (such as lung or breast) in your request.

- *Radiation Therapy and You: A Guide to Self-Help During Treatment.* Radiation therapy, its goals and side effects, and helpful suggestions to patients are discussed in this booklet.

- *Chemotherapy and You: A Guide to Self-Help During Treatment.* This booklet provides detailed information about how chemotherapy is used in cancer treatment and how to manage the side effects of drug treatment.

- *Questions and Answers About Pain Control.* This booklet discusses various medical and nonmedical methods of pain control. It is also available from your local American Cancer Society (see your phone directory for the number to call).

- *Answers to Your Questions About Metastatic Cancer.* This factsheet presents information about what happens when cancer spreads.

■ *Taking Time: Support for People With Cancer and the People Who Care About Them.*
This book discusses the special emotional and personal problems faced by people with cancer.

You can get free, single copies of these and other NCI publications by calling the CIS at 1-800-4-CANCER or by writing to the Office of Cancer Communications, Public Inquiries, NCI, Building 31, Room 10A24, Bethesda, MD 20892.

Support Programs and Organizations

Health professionals and patients have learned the value of mutual support among patients. When someone with a serious illness feels frightened or depressed, it often helps to discuss those feelings with another person who has been through the same experience. This can help patients get practical information, understand their own feelings, and develop ways of handling their problems. Families and other people who are close to someone with a serious illness can also use this type of help.

American Cancer Society

The American Cancer Society (ACS) is a nonprofit organization that offers a variety of services to patients and their families. The ACS sponsors several support groups for patients. Through ACS's CanSurmount Program, for example, people who have recovered from cancer are available to talk with newly diagnosed patients and patients whose cancer has recurred about cancer-related problems and treatments. The ACS also offers the I Can Cope program, which is a course designed to address the educational and psychological needs of people with cancer. Other programs are also available. To find an ACS office near you, check your local telephone book or contact the national office at the following address and telephone number:

American Cancer Society
National Office
1599 Clifton Road, N.E.
Atlanta, GA 30329
404-320-3333

The American Red Cross (ARC) provides instruction in first aid and home nursing. If you need this type of help, your local chapter may be able to help you locate someone to assist with activities such as personal care, housework, and shopping. To receive information about ARC, look in your local phone directory. You may also contact the national office at the following address and telephone number:

American Red Cross
431 18th Street, N.W.
Washington, DC 20006
202-737-8300

Home Health
Care Services

Some patients need home care during or after their cancer treatments. Many state and county health departments have programs that provide instruction in caring for the cancer patient at home. Such knowledge may be very useful after surgery or during illness. Commercial services such as visiting nurse programs may be listed under ''home health agencies'' in your telephone book.

Make Today
Count

This program brings together patients with cancer or other life-threatening illnesses and their families to help them cope with their illnesses and changes in lifestyle that are often required. Support is provided through group meetings, home visit programs, and newsletters. To receive information about this program, contact Make Today Count at the following address and telephone number:

Make Today Count
101 ½ South Union Street
Alexandria, VA 22314
703-548-9674 or 703-548-9714

National Coalition for Cancer Survivorship

The National Coalition for Cancer Survivorship (NCCS) is a network of cancer survivors and related organizatons across the country. It sponsors local support groups for cancer survivors and their families, a national clearinghouse of resources for living with cancer, advocacy to reduce cancer-based discrimination, and a unified voice for cancer survivors. To find a local group of NCCS, contact the national office at the following address and telephone number:

National Coalition for Cancer Survivorship
323 Eighth Street, S.W.
Albuquerque, NM 87102
505-764-9956

The Leukemia Society of America

The Leukemia Society of America offers some financial help and consultation services to cancer patients with leukemia and related disorders. To find out more about the Society, look for a telephone number in your local phone directory. You may also contact the national office:

Leukemia Society of America, Inc.
733 Third Avenue
New York, NY 10017
212-573-8484

The United Ostomy Association

The United Ostomy Association (UOA) is a network of local chapters that offers emotional support, aid, and education to people who have had surgery to create a colostomy, ileostomy, or urostomy. To find a chapter in your area, check the local phone directory under ''ostomy'' or contact the national office at:

United Ostomy Association
Suite 12036 Executive Park
Irvine, CA 92714
714-660-8624

Nutrition for Patients Receiving Chemotherapy and Radiation Treatment, American Cancer Society. Available from local offices of ACS (listed in the telephone book). Contains high-protein, high-calorie recipes for beverages, snacks, and desserts. The recipe for home-blenderized tube feeding is not recommended.

Nutritional Principles and Dietary Guidelines for Patients Receiving Chemotherapy and Radiation Therapy, American Cancer Society. Available from the ACS Milwaukee Division, Inc., 6401 West Capitol Drive, Milwaukee, WI 53216. Discusses the nutritional needs of people receiving chemotherapy or radiation therapy. Includes recommendations for overcoming problems that may affect nutrition such as loss of appetite, food aversions, and nausea. One chapter tells how to change food textures to liquid or semisolid food for persons with chewing or swallowing problems. A list of commercial nutritional supplements is included.

Cooking for the Cancer Patient, Kato Perlman and Jerry Kukachka. Available from the Wisonsin Clinical Cancer Center, Public Affairs Office, 1900 University Avenue, Madison, WI 53706. Features approximately 300 recipes (including blender recipes) designed to meet the nutritional needs of patients with cancer.

Something's Got to Taste Good: The Cancer Patient's Cookbook, J. Fishman, B. Anrod. Available in bookstores or from Andrews and McMeel Publishing Co., 1271 Avenue of Americas, New York 10020, (212) 582-0650. Offers creative, easy recipes and gives protein and calorie information for each. Includes suggestions for increasing protein and calorie levels as well as protein and calorie tables of common foods and fast foods.

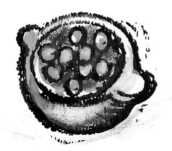

Nutrition and the Cancer Patient, Joyce Daly Margie and Abby S. Bloch. Available at many bookstores and libraries or by contacting Chilson Book Company, Radnor, PA 19089. This self-help book shows the reader how to take an active role during cancer treatment. Several nutrition-related problems and their management are addressed, including caring for children with cancer. Provides more than 300 quick and easy recipes for appetizers, beverages, main entrees, and desserts. Gives names and addresses of groups and organizations throughout the country for both emotional and financial support.

Nutrition for the Cancer Patient, Ernest H. Rosenbaum, Carol N. Stitt, Harry Drasin, and Isadora R. Rosenbaum. Available from Bull Publishing Co., P.O. Box 208, Palo Alto, CA 94302. Discusses possible nutritional problems resulting from cancer or its treatment. Includes suggestions for dealing with these concerns, information on basic nutrition, and 42 pages of recipes. Provides many tips and recipes for dealing with swallowing difficulties.

Blend and Mend, Wilma King. Available from Blend and Mend Publications, P.O. Box 548, Redwood City, CA 94064. Offers high-calorie blender recipes for people on a liquid diet.

Non-Chew Cookbook. Available from Wilson Publishing, Inc., P.O. Box 2190, Glenwood Springs, CO 81602. Contains recipes for patients who are unable to eat solid food because of oral surgery or side effects from radiation therapy or chemotherapy.

The Safe Food Book: Your Kitchen Guide. U.S.D.A. Food Safety and Inspection Service (revised 6/85). Home and Garden Bulletin #241. Available free by calling the U.S.D.A. Meat and Poultry Hotline 1-800-535-4555 (in Washington, D.C., call 447-3333). Gives helpful tips for keeping food safe.

Anorexia: Loss of appetite for food.

Biological therapy: Sometimes called immunotherapy, this treatment uses the body's natural defense system to destroy cancer cells.

Calorie: Calories measure the energy your body gets from food. Your body needs calories as "fuel" to perform all of its functions, such as breathing, circulating the blood, and physical activity. When you are sick, your body may need extra calories to fight fever or other problems.

Carbohydrate: One of the three nutrients that supply calories (energy) to the body. Carbohydrates are needed for normal body function. There are two basic kinds of carbohydrates: simple (sugars) and complex (starches and fiber).

Chemotherapy: The use of drugs to stop cancer cells from growing in size or number.

Dehydration: When the body loses too much water to work well. Severe diarrhea or vomiting can cause dehydration.

Diet: Your diet is the foods you eat, including both liquids and solids.

Dietary fat: One of the three nutrients that supply calories (energy) to the body. Fat also helps the body absorb certain vitamins. Small amounts of fat are necessary for normal body function. Foods high in fat are also high in calories.

Diuretics: Drugs that help the body get rid of water and salt.

Dyspepsia/indigestion: Upset stomach.

Dysphagia: Difficulty in swallowing.

Edema: The buildup of excess fluid within the tissues.

Electrolytes: A general term for the minerals necessary to give the body the proper fluid balance.

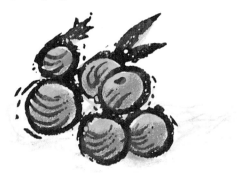

Fortified: A food is fortified when extra nutrients are added.

Glucose: A simple sugar occurring in some fruits and honey; the sugar found in blood.

Infection: When germs enter the body and produce disease, the disease is called an infection. Infections can occur in any part of the body. They cause a fever and other problems, depending on the site of the infection. When the body's natural defense system is strong, it can often fight the entering germs and prevent infection. Cancer treatment can weaken the natural defense system, but good nutrition can help make it stronger.

Intravenous (IV) feeding: When a person receives some of the nutrients he or she needs through a needle in a vein. IV feeding occurs when a person is unable to eat solid food, such as right after surgery.

Lactose intolerance: Lactose is a sugar in milk. After some types of surgery you may no longer be able to digest lactose easily. This lactose intolerance may go away over time. There are special milk products without lactose.

Malnutrition: When the body receives too few of the essential nutrients.

Minerals: Nutrients required by the body in small amounts such as iron, calcium, and potassium.

Nutrient: The part of the food you eat that the body uses to grow, function, and stay alive. The major classes of nutrients that the body needs are proteins, minerals, fats, carbohydrates, and vitamins.

Nutrition: A three-part process that gives the body the nutrients it needs. First, you eat or drink food. Second, the body breaks the food down into nutrients. Third, the nutrients travel through the bloodstream to different parts of the body where they are used as "fuel." To give your body proper nutrition, you have to eat or drink enough of the foods that contain key nutrients.

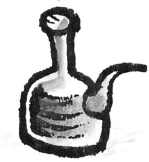

Potassium: A mineral the body needs for fluid balance and other essential functions.

Protein: One of the three nutrients that supply calories (energy) to the body. The protein we eat becomes a part of our muscle, bone, skin, and blood.

Radiation therapy: A cancer treatment that uses high energy rays to destroy the cancer. Also called irradiation, radiotherapy, x-ray therapy.

Sodium: A mineral required by the body to keep body fluids in balance; too much sodium can cause you to retain water.

Total parenteral nutrition (TPN): When a person receives all of the nutrients he or she needs through a needle in a vein. TPN may be used when the mouth, the stomach, or the bowel are sore from cancer treatment.

Vitamins: Key nutrients that the body needs to grow and stay strong. The best source of vitamins, such as vitamins A, B, and C, is the foods we eat.

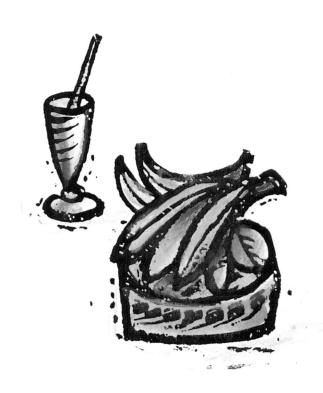

Recipes for Better Nutrition During Cancer Treatment

The recipes were especially chosen to help solve the problems discussed in this book. In order to be included the recipes also had to be high in nutritional value, easy to make, good tasting, and useable for the family as well as for the patient. You will find some old favorites—but calories, protein, or other nutrients have been added. All of the recipes have been taste-tested, and only the favorites from the taste-testing have been included.

At the bottom of each recipe the calories and grams of protein per serving (SV) are indicated. A shaded box indicates that the item is a particularly rich source of calories or protein. The chart also shows which special diets the recipe would be suitable for—a shaded box means that the item is acceptable for the diet listed above it. For example, the Sloppy Joes would be suitable only for the low-lactose diet (see below).

		SPECIAL DIETS			
Calories per SV	Protein g/SV	Full-Liquid	Soft	Low-Residue	Low-Lactose
160	12				▓

Abbreviations: In all recipes, **tsp.** is teaspoon, **tbsp.** is tablespoon, and **lb.** is pound.

Note: No product (brand name listing) endorsement is intended in this book. Brands are named only to insure specific ingredient content, or when a particular brand was consistently acceptable in taste-testing results. Similar products in your own area may work as well, with little or no change in the recipe.

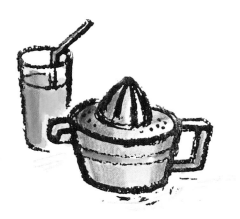

Soft, moist and nourishing, just as popular with or without milk.

Macaroni and Cheese

1 cup milk
1 tbsp. flour
1-2 tbsp. margarine
1 tsp. minced onion

salt and pepper to taste
1 tsp. dry mustard (optional)
2 cups elbow macaroni, cooked
    and drained
1 cup shredded cheddar cheese

Measure milk into the pan and blend in flour until no lumps remain. Add margarine, onion, and other seasonings and cook until sauce thickens. Stir in macaroni and cheese. Bake in greased 1-quart casserole, uncovered, at 400⁰ for 15 minutes, or until slightly browned and bubbly. May be frozen before baking. Serves 4.

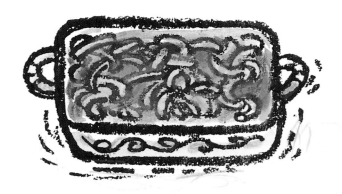

SPECIAL DIETS

Calories per SV	Protein g/SV	Full-Liquid	Soft	Low-Residue	Low-Lactose
275	11			**	*

*Substitute formula for milk, use nondairy margarine and aged cheddar cheese.
**Count milk and cheese as 1¼ cups milk per serving of recipe.

Quickly prepared, this casserole may disappear just as fast at the table!

Cheesy Hamburger Casserole

1 cup macaroni, uncooked
½ lb. ground meat (beef, veal)
½ small onion, chopped

¾ cup tomato sauce or
chopped tomatoes
½ can (10 ounces) cheddar
cheese soup

Cook macaroni until slightly tender. Drain, set aside. Brown ground meat and onions in small skillet. Add tomatoes and simmer 10 minutes. Oil a 1-quart casserole, and spoon in ⅓ of meat mixture. Add cooked macaroni, then the remainder of meat mixture. Spread cheese soup overall (may be frozen, unbaked). Cover the casserole tightly and bake at 400⁰ until bubbly. Makes 4 servings.

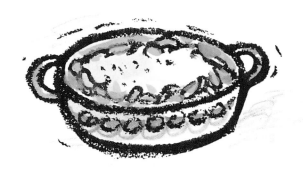

SPECIAL DIETS

Calories per SV	Protein g/SV	Full-Liquid	Soft	Low-Residue	Low-Lactose
215	16				*

*Omit cheese soup, add ½ cup water and 2 ozs. aged cheddar cheese.

This is a simple one-dish meal, a cousin to Quiche Lorraine. Just the thing for a night when you don't want to fuss.

Cheese-Spinach Pie

⅓ cup chopped onion
1 tbsp. margarine
¼ lb. sliced cheese (Swiss or muenster)
1 cup cooked, chopped spinach (drained)

3 large eggs
⅓-½ cup of milk
½ tsp. salt
dash pepper
9-inch pie shell

Cook onion in margarine until tender; cool. Lay slices of cheese over pie dough, follow with spinach, then onions. Beat eggs, adding enough milk to make 1 cup. Add seasonings and pour over ingredients in the pie shell. Bake in 400° oven about 35 minutes, or until a knife comes out clean. Serve piping hot. (Can be frozen after baking.) Serves 4.

Variation: Substitute cooked, chopped broccoli, green beans, zucchini, or peas for spinach.

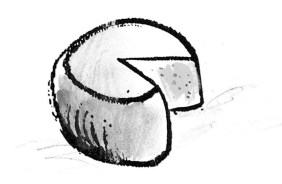

SPECIAL DIETS

Calories per SV	Protein g/SV	Full-Liquid	Soft	Low-Residue	Low-Lactose
454	18				*

*Substitute soy formula for milk. Use nondairy margarine and aged natural cheese and milk-free dough.

56

A reliable, mildly flavored recipe which can adapt to your needs.

Basic Meatloaf or Meatballs

2 tbsp. dry bread or cracker
  crumbs
1 tbsp. water
½ lb. ground beef or veal
1 egg

¼ tsp. minced onion
salt and pepper to taste
1 tbsp. oil or margarine
2 slices onion

Combine crumbs and water in small mixing bowl. Add meat, minced onion, egg, and seasonings. Mix until well-blended. Form into patties, 1-inch meatballs, or a loaf. Brown in oil or margarine in skillet, turn to brown both sides. Add sliced onion, lower heat, cover and simmer for at least 15 minutes, 30 minutes for meatloaf. You can also bake at 350⁰. For meatballs, bake 30 minutes, turning after 15 minutes. For meatloaf, bake 1 hour. Can be frozen raw or cooked. Makes 4 servings.

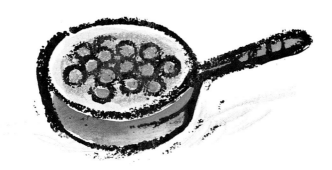

SPECIAL DIETS

Calories per SV	Protein g/SV	Full-Liquid	Soft	Low-Residue	Low-Lactose
125	13				*

*Use milk-free bread crumbs.

Sloppy Joes

½ lb. ground meat   ½ cup quick barbecue sauce
1 small onion, diced   1 tbsp. raw oatmeal

Brown meat and onion in skillet. Add barbecue sauce, oatmeal, and enough water to cover meat. Heat to boiling, turn down heat to simmer, cover pan, and cook 15 minutes or until thickened and meat is soft. Serve on buns, toast, or hard rolls. Can be frozen after cooking. Serves 4.

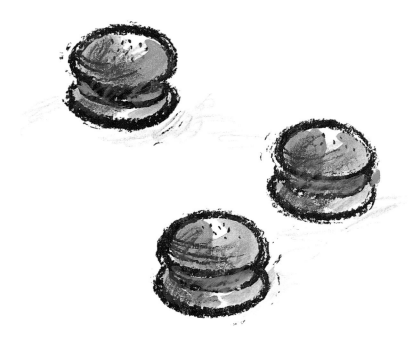

| | | SPECIAL DIETS | | | |
Calories per SV	Protein g/SV	Full-Liquid	Soft	Low-Residue	Low-Lactose
160	12				

These are tender meatballs with gourmet flavor.

Swedish Meatballs

1 lb. ground round steak	⅔ tsp. salt
½ cup plain bread crumbs	dash pepper and allspice
1 egg, slightly beaten	1 tbsp. margarine

Mix all ingredients except margarine with a fork until well blended. Form into balls, brown in margarine in medium-sized skillet. Remove meatballs from pan. Make a thickened gravy with the drippings. Return meatballs to gravy and simmer, covered, for 1 to 1½ hours. May be frozen raw or cooked. Serves 4.

Contributed by D. Ruth Gilbert.

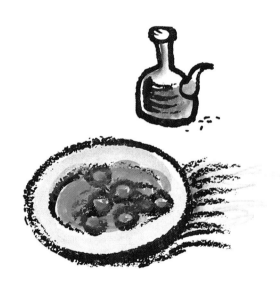

		SPECIAL DIETS			
Calories per SV	Protein g/SV	Full-Liquid	Soft	Low-Residue	Low-Lactose
281	25				*

*Use milk-free bread crumbs.

Supremely simple to make, this is a delightfully seasoned entree.

Chicken Supreme

1 can (10 ozs.) cream of
   mushroom soup
½ cup orange juice
½ cup water

1 cup rice, uncooked
6 pieces chicken
¼ envelope onion soup mix

Combine first four ingredients and pour into greased 2-quart casserole. Lay chicken on top. Sprinkle with dry onion soup mix. Cover casserole, airtight, with heavy aluminum foil. Bake 2 hours without opening the foil, at 350°. Can be frozen after baking. Serves 6.

Contributed by a patient.

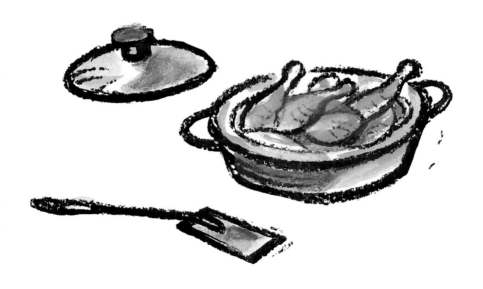

SPECIAL DIETS

Calories per SV	Protein g/SV	Full-Liquid	Soft	Low-Residue	Low-Lactose
295	18				

Tender and lightly seasoned, this simple dish can be a complete meal with rice, noodles, or mashed potatoes.

Chicken Skillet Supper

2-3 lbs. frying chicken, cut up
½ can (10 oz.) vegetarian-
   vegetable soup

1 can water
2 sprigs of parsley
1 basil leaf (optional)

Place chicken, skin side down, in cold skillet. Brown over medium heat, turning to brown inside. Remove from heat (chicken skin can easily be removed at this point if you wish). Pour off all fat remaining in skillet. Replace chicken, pour soup and water over chicken, and add seasonings. Simmer 1 hour in covered skillet, turning pieces once to keep them moist. May be frozen after cooking. Serves 4.

Tomato special: Substitute ½ can of cream of tomato for vegetarian-vegetable soup. Add 1 package (10 oz.) of mixed frozen vegetables with the soup and water.

Creamy chicken: Substitute ½ can of cream of chicken for vegetarian-vegetable soup, add 1 package (10 oz.) frozen peas and carrots.

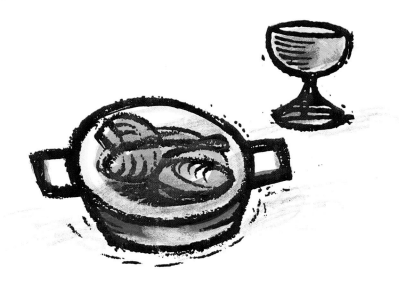

Calories per SV	Protein g/SV	SPECIAL DIETS			
		Full-Liquid	Soft	Low-Residue	Low-Lactose
200	24				

This mild flavored tuna dish is complemented with a tossed salad.

Robert's Tuna Bake

1 can (7 oz.) water-packed
  tuna, broken in small pieces
1 can (10 oz.) tomato soup
½ cup milk

¼ lb. American or cheddar
  cheese
1 lb. box of elbow macaroni,
  cooked

Mix first four ingredients in saucepan and heat until cheese melts. Add macaroni to sauce and mix well. Pour into greased baking dish and bake at 350⁰ for 20 minutes. Serves 8.

Chicken Noodle Bake: Substitute cream of celery soup for tomato, 1 cup diced chicken for tuna, cooked noodles for elbow macaroni.

Egg Noodle Bake: Substitute cream of chicken soup for tomato, 3 or more sliced hard-boiled eggs, for tuna, and cooked noodles for elbow macaroni.

Contributed by Mr. Robert L. Card.

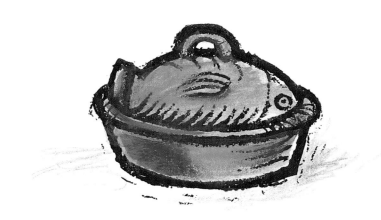

SPECIAL DIETS

Calories per SV	Protein g/SV	Full-Liquid	Soft	Low-Residue	Low-Lactose
435	24			**	*

*Substitute soy formula for milk. Use aged cheddar cheese.
**Count cheese as ½ cup milk.

A surprising balance of flavors will please busy cooks and their families.

Tuna Broccoli Casserole

2 packages (10 ozs.) frozen broccoli, whole or chopped
2 cans (7 ozs.) water-packed tuna broken in small pieces
1 can (10 ozs.) cream of mushroom soup diluted with ½ cup of milk
1 cup grated cheddar or American cheese
½ cup plain bread crumbs
2 tbsp. melted margarine

Cook broccoli according to package directions, drain, and place in shallow 2-quart casserole. Add tuna and cover with diluted mushroom soup. Sprinkle with cheese. Add bread crumbs to melted butter and sprinkle over casserole. Bake at 350⁰ for 20 minutes. Serves 5.

Contributed by a patient.

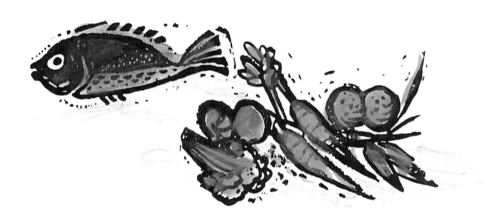

SPECIAL DIETS

Calories per SV	Protein g/SV	Full-Liquid	Soft	Low-Residue	Low-Lactose
290	25				*

*Substitute aged cheddar cheese, nondairy margarine, and use water instead of milk.

A light potato salad, mildly seasoned for the sensitive palate.

Creamy Potato Salad

⅓ cup plain low-fat yogurt
⅓ cup mayonnaise
¼ tsp. finely minced or
  scraped onion
1 sprig of parsley, finely
  chopped

¼ cup chopped celery or green
  pepper (optional)
2 potatoes, boiled and diced
2 hard-boiled eggs, diced
salt to taste

Blend yogurt, mayonnaise, onion, parsley, celery, and pepper. Stir in remaining ingredients. Cover and refrigerate for several hours. Serves 4.

Ricotta Potato Salad: Add ⅓ cup ricotta cheese to mayonnaise.

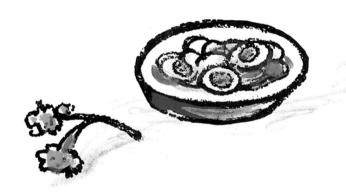

SPECIAL DIETS

Calories per SV	Protein g/SV	Full-Liquid	Soft	Low-Residue	Low-Lactose
245	5		**		*

*Use yogurt made only from cultured pasteurized milk.
**Omit onion, celery, green pepper.

A quick, flavorful sauce everybody enjoys on eggs or meat.

Creole Sauce

½ small onion, sliced
1 or 2 frying peppers (1 bell
    pepper) cleaned and sliced
2 tbsp. oil
2 cups chopped fresh
    tomatoes or 15 ounce can
    of tomatoes

½ tsp. salt
2 tbsp. sugar
1 tsp. vinegar
1 tbsp. cornstarch
water

Fry onion and peppers in oil until onion is clear and pepper is spotted with brown. Add tomatoes, salt, sugar, and vinegar. Bring to boiling, turn down to simmer. Cover and cook at least 20 minutes to blend the flavors. Thicken just before serving with cornstarch dissolved in a little water. Use on eggs or meat. Makes 2 cups (½ cup = 1 serving).

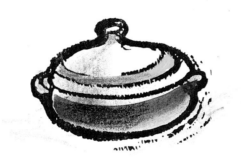

SPECIAL DIETS

Calories per SV	Protein g/SV	Full-Liquid	Soft	Low-Residue	Low-Lactose
150	2				

Quick Barbecue Sauce

½ cup catsup
2 tsps. salad style mustard
½ tsp. lemon juice

1 tbsp. brown sugar
½ tsp. onion salt

Mix together in small saucepan. Heat until boiling, stirring as it cooks.

Serving suggestions: Make Sloppy Joes. Use as a barbecue sauce for hot dogs, chicken, or meatballs. (It will easily coat eight pieces of chicken.) Use as a marinade for chicken or meat: pour over pieces in a deep dish, and refrigerate in marinade, at least 12 hours to tenderize. Makes ½ cup.

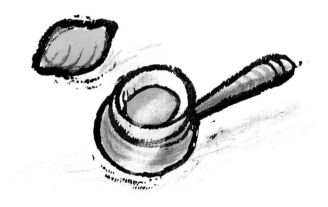

		SPECIAL DIETS			
Calories per recipe	Protein per recipe	Full-Liquid	Soft	Low-Residue	Low-Lactose
208	2				

An unexpected favorite. This tangy sauce is often used on meat or chicken.

Sweet and Sour Sauce

¼ cup vinegar
1 cup catsup
1 tbsp. soy sauce
½ red or green pepper, cubed
½ cup honey or brown sugar
  (packed)

½ tsp. salt
1 can (8 ounce size) pineapple
  chunks (optional)
water
2 tbsp. cornstarch

Mix all ingredients except cornstarch in saucepan. Bring to boil. Turn heat down to simmer, stirring occasionally and cook for at least 20 minutes to allow flavors to blend. Dissolve cornstarch in small amount of water. Add, stirring until thickened. (You can omit cornstarch and allow the sauce to thicken by cooking it longer.) Use on meat or chicken. Makes 2 cups.

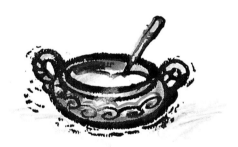

SPECIAL DIETS

Calories per cup	Protein g/cup	Full-Liquid	Soft	Low-Residue	Low-Lactose
590	3				

These pancakes have double the protein of regular pancakes. Two of them equal 1 ounce of meat in protein content.

High-Protein Pancakes

½ cup milk
2 tbsp. dry milk
1 egg (2 for a thinner crepe-type)

2 tsps. of oil
½-¾ cups pancake mix

Measure milk, dry milk, egg, and oil into blender or bowl. Beat until egg is well blended. Add pancake mix. Stir or blend at low speed until mix is wet but some lumps remain. Cook on hot greased griddle or fry pan, turning when firm to brown the other side. These can be kept warm in a warm oven, or in a covered pan on low heat. Makes seven 4'' pancakes.

Note: If there is batter left over, it will keep 1 day in the refrigerator, or it can be made into pancakes, cooled, and wrapped in foil to be frozen for later use. To reheat, leave in foil and place in 450⁰ oven for 15 minutes. If using a toaster oven, unwrap them, brush with margarine, and toast as for light toast.

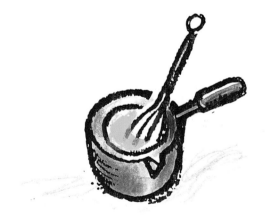

SPECIAL DIETS

Calories per pancake	Protein per pancake	Full-Liquid	Soft	Low-Residue	Low-Lactose
77	3			*	

* Count milk as part of 2 cup limit.

These pancakes have the high protein quality without a drop of milk.

Low-Lactose Pancakes

1 egg (2 for crepe-type)
½ cup soy formula

2 tsps. milk-free margarine,
 melted
½ cup milk-free pancake mix*

Into bowl or blender put egg, soy formula, and melted margarine. Beat to blend. Stir in mix until wet but some lumps remain. Cook on greased or oiled pan (use only milk-free margarine, bacon fat, or shortening) until firm enough to turn over. Brown other side. Keep warm in oven or in covered pan on low heat. If you wish to freeze pancakes, follow directions in recipe for High-Protein Pancakes. Makes six 4'' pancakes.

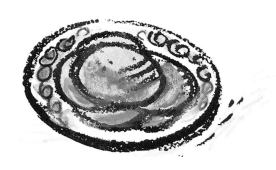

SPECIAL DIETS

Calories per pancake	Protein per pancake	Full-Liquid	Soft	Low-Residue	Low-Lactose
88	2				

*Pillsbury's Hungry Jack Extra Lights is a lactose-free mix. Aunt Jemima's Whole Wheat may contain a small amount of lactose.

Doubles the protein in each cup of milk. Used in many recipes in this booklet.

Fortified Milk

1 quart milk, homogenized   1 cup instant nonfat dry milk
or 1% low-fat

Pour liquid milk into deep bowl. Add dry milk and beat slowly with beater until dry milk is dissolved (usually less than 5 minutes). Refrigerate. The flavor improves after several hours. Makes 1 quart.

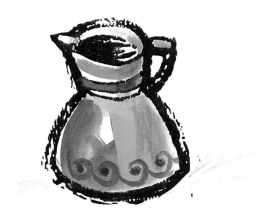

| | | SPECIAL DIETS | | | |
Calories per cup	Protein g/cup	Full-Liquid	Soft	Low-Residue	Low-Lactose
WHOLE MILK					
275	19				
1% MILK					
195	19				

A tasty banana shake is a rich potassium source.

Vera's Banana Milkshake

1 whole ripe banana, sliced   vanilla (few drops)
1 cup milk

Measure into blender and blend at high speed until smooth. Serves 1.

Banana-butterscotch: Add 2 tbsp. of butterscotch sauce with banana.

Contributed by Vera Bagley.

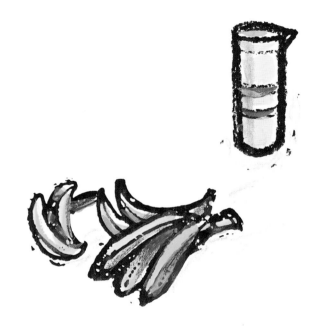

SPECIAL DIETS

Calories per SV	Protein g/SV	Full-Liquid	Soft	Low-Residue	Low-Lactose
275	9			**	*

*Substitute soy formula for milk.
**Count as half of 2 cups allowed milk per day.

The flavor of fresh strawberries, but from the freezer.

Pearl's Strawberry Milkshake

½ cup frozen strawberries
1 scoop ice cream
½ cup milk

Mix or blend until smooth. Serves 1.

Contributed by Pearl L. Howard.

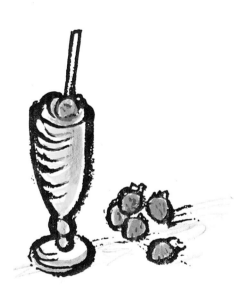

SPECIAL DIETS

Calories per SV	Protein g/SV	Full-Liquid	Soft	Low-Residue	Low-Lactose
355	7			*	

*Count as half of 2 cup daily milk allowance.

Favorite milkshake flavors with extra protein.

High-Protein Milkshakes

1 cup fortified milk
1 generous scoop ice cream
½ tsp. vanilla

2 tbsp. of butterscotch,
  chocolate, or your favorite
  fruit syrup or sauce

Measure all ingredients into blender. Blend at low speed about 10 seconds. Makes 1 serving.

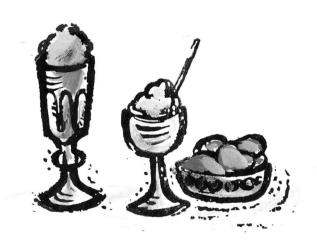

		SPECIAL DIETS			
Calories per SV	Protein g/SV	Full-Liquid	Soft	Low-Residue	Low-Lactose
485	22				

Citrus Fake Shakes

1 frozen citrus fruit juice bar (2½ ozs.) or 2 bars (1¾ ozs.) same flavor
½ cup chilled Isomil or Neomullsoy
¼ tsp. vanilla

Remove citrus bar from freezer and allow to thaw slightly (about 5-10 minutes until soft). Break bar into pieces into blender. Add other ingredients and blend at low speed for 10 seconds. Makes 1 serving.

Double citrus: You can increase the use of orange juice without drinking it by adding 1 tbsp. frozen orange juice concentrate and 1 tbsp. sugar to the lemon or orange flavor Fake Shake before blending.

		SPECIAL DIETS			
Calories per cup	Protein g/cup	Full-Liquid	Soft	Low-Residue	Low-Lactose
CITRUS					
114	3	■	■	■	■
BUTTERSCOTCH					
222	3	■	■	■	*
CHOCOLATE					
165	3	■	■	■	■
BUTTERSCOTCH BANANA					
274	3		■	■	*
PEANUT BUTTER-HONEY					
255	13		■		
FAKE SHAKE SHERBET					
255	13		■		

*Use milk-free butterscotch sauce.

Other Fake Shakes

Butterscotch

½ cup chilled or partially frozen Isomil or Neomullsoy
¼ tsp. vanilla
2 tbsp. milk-free butterscotch sauce

Blend all at low speed about 10 seconds. Using the partially frozen liquid will produce a much colder, thicker shake. Makes 1 serving.

Chocolate

Use 2 tbsp. Hershey's chocolate syrup in place of butterscotch. (Commercial chocolate syrups are often made without milk or lactose, but always read the ingredient labels.)

Butterscotch Banana

Add ½ well ripened, sliced banana to ingredients for butterscotch shake.

Peanut Butter-Honey

Omit butterscotch sauce. Mix together in a cup: ¼ cup soy formula or nondairy creamer, 2 tbsp. smooth peanut butter, 1 tbsp. honey, and ¼ tsp. vanilla. Place partially frozen liquid in blender, then add peanut butter mixture. Blend for about 10 seconds, or until smooth.

Fake Shake Sherbet

Follow recipe for Peanut Butter-Honey above (you can double or triple recipe easily to save time). Pour shake into small container. Freeze 2 hours or until it begins to harden around edges. Scrape into bowl and mix thoroughly, until lumps disappear. Return to container and refreeze 2 hours or until firm.

Fake Shake Ice Cream

Any of the shakes above can be frozen into ice creams, using the same method as for Fake Shake Sherbet.

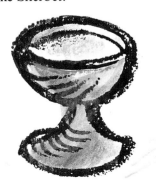

An occasional drink has helped boost many a lagging appetite. It is important to know whether your physician allows alcohol before you sample the enriched drinks.

Fruit Smoothie

2 tbsp. blackberry or cherry cordial

¾ cup chilled or partially frozen half-and-half

Mix or blend until smooth. Serve in a fancy glass frosted, if you like. Serves 1.

Panamanian Smoothie
Omit cordial; add 2 tbsp. chocolate syrup and 2 tbsp. rum.

Creme de Menthe Smoothie
Omit cordial; add 2 tbsp. creme de menthe and 2 tbsp. vanilla ice cream (omit ice cream for low-lactose).

| | | SPECIAL DIETS | | | |
Calories per SV	Protein g/SV	Full-Liquid	Soft	Low-Residue	Low-Lactose
FRUIT					
295	5			**	*
PANAMANIAN					
400	6			**	*
CREME DE MENTHE					
330	6			**	*

*Substitute nondairy creamer and omit ice cream. The cordials do not contain lactose.
**Count half-and-half as part of 2 cups milk allowed per day.

Amaretto Creme

½ cup chilled half-and-half   1 tbsp. Amaretto cordial
2 tbsp. vanilla ice cream

Mix until smooth. Serve in stemmed glass. Serves 1.

Butterscotch Brandy Creme
Omit Amaretto; add 2 tbsp. butterscotch sauce and 1 tbsp. brandy.

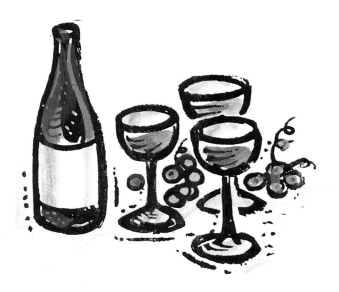

Calories per SV	Protein g/SV	SPECIAL DIETS			
		Full-Liquid	Soft	Low-Residue	Low-Lactose
245	4			**	*

*Substitute nondairy creamer and omit ice cream (Amaretto).
 Substitute nondairy creamer and milk-free butterscotch sauce
 (Butterscotch Brandy Creme).
**Count half-and-half and ice cream as part of 2 cups milk allowed per day.

The sweet-tart taste of this sauce is a change from sweet syrup. Good on pancakes and waffles.

Fresh Peach Sauce

1 large peach, peeled and thinly sliced 1½ tbsp. sugar	¼ cup water 1 tsp. cornstarch dash nutmeg

Combine ingredients in a small pan, stir until cornstarch is dissolved. Cook over medium heat until sauce boils and is thickened. Serves 1.

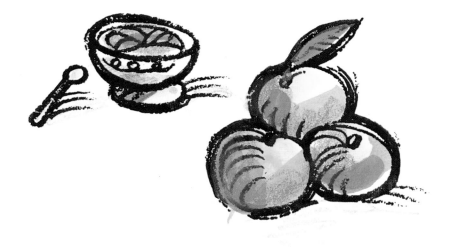

SPECIAL DIETS

Calories per SV	Protein g/SV	Full- Liquid	Soft	Low- Residue	Low- Lactose
140	0				

This tasty sauce is good for many toppings.

Milk-Free Butterscotch Sauce

⅓ cup brown sugar, packed
2 tsp. cornstarch
¼ cup nondairy creamer

¼ cup water
1 tbsp. honey
1 tbsp. milk-free margarine
½ tsp. vanilla

Mix brown sugar and cornstarch in small saucepan. Slowly add nondairy creamer and water, stirring until cornstarch dissolves. Add honey and margarine. Cook over medium heat, stirring constantly, until sauce is thickened and comes to a boil. Remove from heat. Add vanilla. Cook and store in a covered container in refrigerator. Makes about ½ cup.

Milk-Free Chocolate: Stir in 1 heaping tbsp. cocoa with cornstarch. If too thick, add a little water after it comes to a boil.

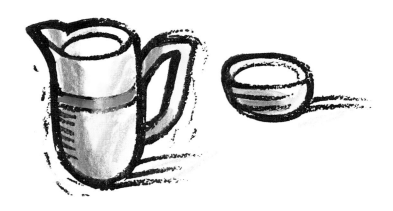

SPECIAL DIETS

Calories per tbsp.	Protein g/tbsp.	Full-Liquid	Soft	Low-Residue	Low-Lactose
85	0				

A high-protein snack of good quality—the milk protein balanced by the peanut protein.

Peanut Butter Snack Spread

1 tbsp. instant dry milk
1 tsp. water
1 tsp. vanilla

1 tbsp. honey
3 heaping tbsp. creamy
  peanut butter

Combine dry milk, water, and vanilla, stirring to moisten. Add honey and peanut butter, stirring slowly until liquid begins to blend with peanut butter. Spread between graham crackers or milk lunch crackers. The spread can also be formed into balls, chilled, and eaten as candy. Keeps well in refrigerator, but is difficult to spread when cold. Makes ⅓ cup.

Molasses Taffy Flavor: Substitute molasses for honey.

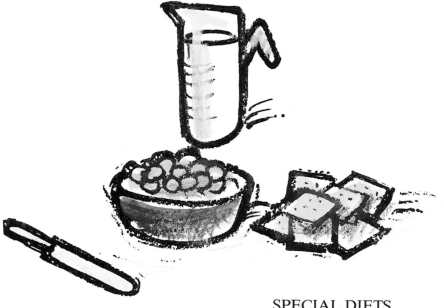

SPECIAL DIETS

Calories per SV	Protein g/SV	Full-Liquid	Soft	Low-Residue	Low-Lactose
440	17			**	*

*Substitute 1 tbsp. soy formula for milk and water.
**Count dry milk as ¼ cup milk of 2 cups allowed per day.

This natural fiber snack or cereal comes with the nutrition of milk. It can also be made without milk.

Granola I

1½ cups quick oatmeal
½ cup regular wheat germ
½ cup coconut
½ tsp. salt

½ cup chopped nuts
2 tbsp. oil
⅔ cup sweetened condensed milk

Measure oatmeal, wheat germ, coconut, salt, and nuts into mixing bowl, stirring to blend. Add oil and mix thoroughly. Pour in condensed milk and blend well. Sprinkle a handful of wheat germ on a cookie sheet and gently spread mixture on top. Bake in 325⁰ oven, about 25 minutes. Check mix as it bakes—after the first 10 minutes, mix will begin to brown. Stir it on cookie sheet every 10 minutes until it is as brown as you like. Cool on pan; store in covered container in refrigerator.

Granola II: Omit milk. Add ½ cup honey. Bake as above.

Chocolate chip: Put hot mixture in bowl. Stir in ½ cup of chocolate chips.

Raisin: Stir in 1 cup of raisins after the mixture cools.

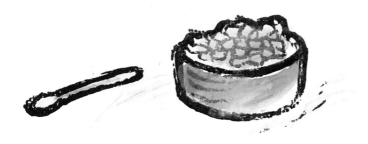

SPECIAL DIETS

Calories per ½ cup	Protein per ½ cup	Full-Liquid	Soft	Low-Residue	Low-Lactose
GRANOLA I					
330	9				
GRANOLA II					
340	7				

A chewy, delightful bar. Great with tea or for a snack for the children with milk.

Granola Bars

¾ cup quick cooking oatmeal
½ cup Granola II
½ cup coconut
½ cup brown sugar (packed)
¼ cup melted margarine

1 egg
¼ tsp. vanilla extract
1 tbsp. honey
¼ tsp. salt
¼ cup flour

Measure oatmeal, granola, coconut, and brown sugar together in deep bowl. Mix well. Pour melted margarine over all and blend thoroughly. Beat the egg, extract, honey, and salt together. Pour this over dry ingredients, stirring to blend. Add flour, stirring until smoothly mixed. Press mixture onto greased, floured 11x7-inch shallow baking pan or cookie sheet. Bake at 325⁰ for 35 minutes. Cool slightly, cut into bars, and remove from the pan while warm. Makes 18 bars.

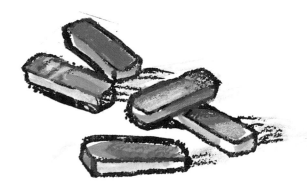

SPECIAL DIETS

Calories per bar	Protein per bar	Full-Liquid	Soft	Low-Residue	Low-Lactose
60	2				

A soft, delightful dessert made with bread and tasty apples.

Apple Brown Betty

4 cups thinly sliced pared apples or
  1 can (16 oz.) pie apples,
  drained
2 cups bread cubes or torn
  bread pieces
½ cup brown sugar, packed

$1/8$ tsp. ground cinnamon
2 tbsp. margarine
¼ cup hot water

Grease 1-quart baking dish. Arrange half of apples on bottom of dish. Follow with half of bread, then half of sugar. Repeat layers. Sprinkle cinnamon over top, cut margarine in pieces and lay them on top, finish by pouring hot water over all. Cover and bake at 350⁰ for 30 minutes, uncover and bake 10 minutes longer. Serve warm or chilled. Serves 4.

Apple Cheese Betty: Spoon 1 cup ricotta cheese over first layer of apples, bread, and sugar. Complete as above.

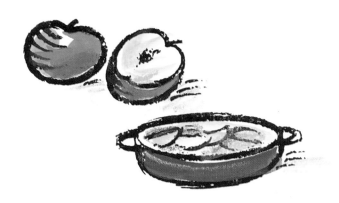

SPECIAL DIETS

Calories per cup	Protein g/cup	Full-Liquid	Soft	Low-Residue	Low-Lactose
WITHOUT CHEESE					
291	1			*	
WITH CHEESE					
342	4			**	

*Count apples as 2 servings fruit (maximum allowed per day).
**Count apples as above and ¼ cup cheese as 1 cup of milk.

Delightful as a plain moist cake, or mouth-watering when iced with Helen's chocolate frosting.

Adair's Apple Raisin Cake

1¾ cup coarsely chopped
   apples, or drained canned
   pie apples, chopped
¾ cup brown sugar, packed
½ cup oil
1 egg, beaten
½ tsp. baking soda
1 tsp. baking powder

½ tsp. salt
1½ cups flour
1 tsp. cinnamon
½ tsp. nutmeg
½ cup raisins, plumped in
   warm water
½ cup chopped nuts

Measure apples and brown sugar into bowl. Add oil and eggs. Add dry ingredients and mix well. This dough will be stiff.

Add raisins and nuts. Stir to blend. Spread in 8-inch square pan. Bake at 350⁰ for 40 minutes or until top springs back when touched. May be frozen. Makes 16 pieces.

Contributed by Adair Luciani.

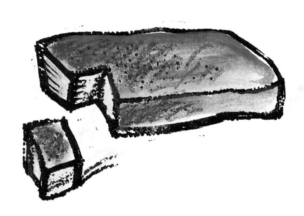

Calories per piece	Protein per piece	SPECIAL DIETS			
		Full-Liquid	Soft	Low-Residue	Low-Lactose
200	3				

Individual Cheese Pies

1 tbsp. ricotta cheese
1 tbsp. applesauce (pureed),
  peaches, or drained crushed
  pineapple

2 tsp. sugar
sprinkle of cinnamon
one 3-inch sugar cookie
  (store bought)

Blend cheese, fruit, sugar, and cinnamon. Spoon over a sugar cookie, turned upside down so the sugar side is on the bottom next to the cookie sheet or foil. Bake at 350⁰ for 15 minutes (the cookie softens as it absorbs the liquid from the fruit-cheese mixture; for a softer treat, lower the oven to 325⁰). Serves 1.

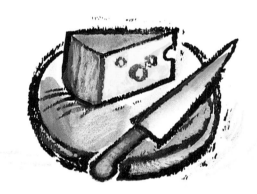

| | | | SPECIAL DIETS | | |
Calories per pie	Protein per pie	Full-Liquid	Soft	Low-Residue	Low-Lactose
85	2			*	

*Count cheese towards 2 cups of milk allowed per day.

A quickly made bread, high on the list of nourishing foods.

Banana-Nut Bread

2 eggs
3 medium well-ripened
   bananas, cut into chunks
¼ cup of milk
¼ cup of oil
1 tsp. vanilla extract
2 cups all-purpose flour

¾ cup sugar
1 tbsp. baking powder
½ tsp. baking soda
½ tsp. salt
¼ tsp. nutmeg
½-1 cup chopped walnuts or
   pecans, or wheat germ

Blend eggs, bananas, milk, oil, and vanilla at medium speed until smooth, about 15 seconds. Measure rest of ingredients into bowl and stir to mix. Make a well in the center of the dry ingredients and pour in banana mixture. Mix just enough to moisten. Add nuts. Spread batter into well greased 9x5x3-inch loaf pan or three small 5x3x2-inch pans. Bake the bread at 350°, about 1 hour for the large loaf and 35-45 minutes for the smaller ones. Makes 1 large loaf or 3 small loaves (16 slices).

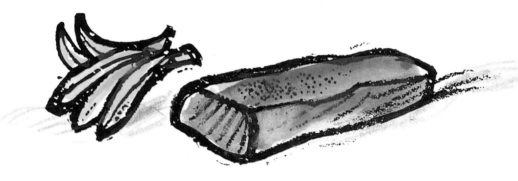

SPECIAL DIETS

Calories per SV	Protein g/SV	Full-Liquid	Soft	Low-Residue	Low-Lactose
185	3				*

*Omit milk, use nondairy creamer or soy formula.

A good, fast-cooked icing.

Helen's Soft Chocolate Frosting

½ cup white sugar
½ cup brown sugar
3 heaping tbsp. cocoa
3 heaping tbsp. cornstarch

1 cup milk
3 tbsp. margarine

Mix first four ingredients together in saucepan until well blended. Gradually add milk. Add margarine. Cook over medium heat, stirring constantly until thick and smooth. (You may need to remove from heat occasionally to prevent sticking or lumping.) Ice cake while the frosting is still warm. Ices two 9-inch layers (serving 16 people). Recipe can easily be cut in half for a single layer cake or cupcakes.

Contributed by Helen Monahan.

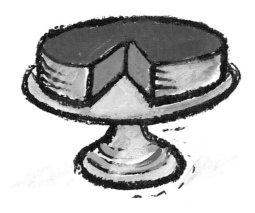

		SPECIAL DIETS			
Calories per SV	Protein g/SV	Full-Liquid	Soft	Low-Residue	Low-Lactose
91	1				*

*Substitute water for milk. Use nondairy margarine.

Cowboy Cookies

1 cup soft shortening or
   margarine
¾ cup brown sugar, packed
¾ cup granulated sugar
2 eggs
1 tsp. vanilla extract
2 cups flour
½ tsp. baking soda

½ tsp. salt
1½ cups quick cooking oatmeal
½ cup coarsely chopped nuts
   or wheat germ
6 ozs. chocolate chips
1 cup raisins

Cream shortening, add sugars, and beat well. Add the eggs and vanilla
and stir to blend well. Add the dry ingredients at one time. Mix to blend
thoroughly. Last, stir in oatmeal, nuts, chocolate chips, and raisins. Mix
well. Drop by spoonfuls on cookie sheet and bake for 13-15 minutes in
350⁰ oven. This dough freezes well and can be sliced later to make fresh
cookies. Makes 4 dozen large cookies.

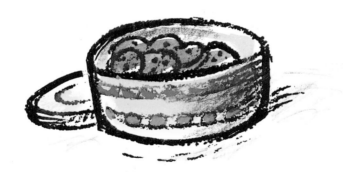

SPECIAL DIETS

Calories per cookie	Protein per cookie	Full-Liquid	Soft	Low-Residue	Low-Lactose
135	2				

Peanut butter fans will like this nourishing bar cookie.

Peanut Butter Bars

¼ cup margarine
¼ cup smooth peanut butter
1⅓ cups brown sugar, packed
2 eggs

1½ cups flour
1½ tsp. baking powder
½ cup chocolate chips
½ cup finely chopped nuts
(optional)

Cream margarine and peanut butter. Add brown sugar and mix well. Add both eggs and mix until well blended. Stir in dry ingredients until blended, then chocolate chips and nuts. Spread batter in greased and floured 9-inch square pan. Bake at 350° for 30-35 minutes. Cool in pan. Cut when cooled into 36 bars.

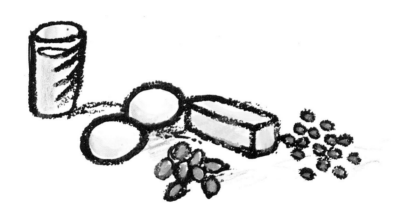

SPECIAL DIETS

Calories per bar	Protein per bar	Full-Liquid	Soft	Low-Residue	Low-Lactose
90	2		*		

*Omit nuts.

Fluffy Fruit Gelatin

1 cup cooked or canned peaches with syrup
1 package red gelatin (3 ozs.)
1 cup boiling water

Blend fruit with syrup at high speed until smooth. Pour pureed fruit back into measuring cup and add enough syrup or water to make one cup. Dissolve gelatin in boiling water, pour into a bowl (deep enough to whip gelatin later). Stir in fruit puree. Cool. Refrigerate gelatin mixture until it piles softly, but is not firm. With cold beaters, whip the gelatin until foamy and doubled in volume. Refrigerate until firm. Serves 6.

Other fruits: Use pears, applesauce, or apricots in place of peaches.

Fluffy Fruit Cream: Fold in 1 cup of whipped cream or nondairy whipped topping after whipping the gelatin. Refrigerate until firm.

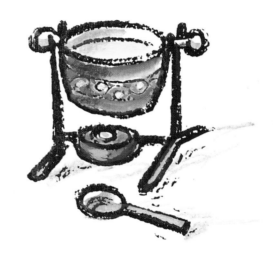

		SPECIAL DIETS			
Calories per SV	Protein g/SV	Full-Liquid	Soft	Low-Residue	Low-Lactose
90	1			*	

*Count as 1 serving of fruit out of daily allowance.

An old standby which is still popular. Serve it hot or chilled.

Rice Pudding

1 tbsp. cornstarch	1 cup milk
1½ tbsp. granulated sugar	½ cup well cooked rice
1 beaten egg	½ tsp. vanilla

Blend first three ingredients in saucepan until smooth. Add milk slowly, stirring to mix well. Add rice. Cook over medium heat, stirring constantly until mixture is thickened and comes to a boil. Remove from heat, add vanilla, and cool. Sprinkle with cinnamon and nutmeg if desired. Many prefer rice pudding warm. Try it for a new taste treat. Makes 3 servings.

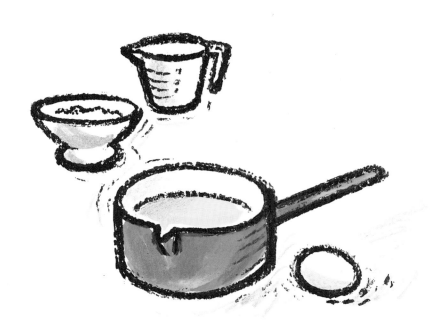

SPECIAL DIETS

Calories per SV	Protein g/SV	Full-Liquid	Soft	Low-Residue	Low-Lactose
140	6			**	*

*Substitute soy formula for milk.
**Count milk towards 2 cups allowed per day.

Milk-Free Double Chocolate Pudding

2 squares baking chocolate
  (1 oz. each)
1 tbsp. cornstarch

¼ cup granulated sugar
1 cup nondairy creamer or
  soy formula
1 tsp. vanilla

Melt chocolate in small pan or on foil. Measure cornstarch and sugar into saucepan. Add part of the creamer and stir until cornstarch dissolves. Add the remainder of the creamer. Cook over medium heat until warm. Stir in chocolate until mixture is thick and comes to a boil. Remove from heat. Blend in vanilla and cool. Makes 2 servings.

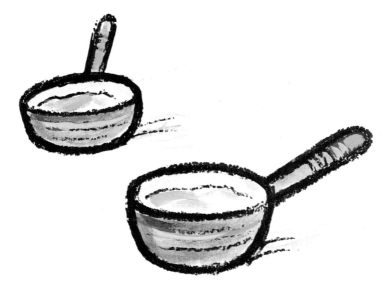

SPECIAL DIETS

Calories per SV	Protein g/SV	Full-Liquid	Soft	Low-Residue	Low-Lactose
WITH SOY FORMULA					
370	11				
WITH NONDAIRY CREAMER					
455	5				

A pleasant dessert for those with a "sweet tooth" who cannot drink milk.

Milk-Free Vanilla Pudding

¼ cup sugar

2 tbsp. cornstarch

2 cups Isomil or Neomullsoy

1 egg, beaten

1 tsp. vanilla

Measure sugar and cornstarch into saucepan. Add a little of the soy formula. Stir to dissolve cornstarch, then pour in the rest of the liquid. Add beaten egg. Cook over medium heat until it comes to a boil and is thickened. Add vanilla and cool. Makes 4 servings.

Maple Pudding: Omit vanilla and add ½ tsp. maple flavoring.

Maple-Nut Pudding: Add ¼ to ½ cup chopped walnuts or pecans to cooled pudding. (Not permitted on soft diet).

Coconut Pudding: Add ½ cup coconut. Read the ingredient listing on coconut to be sure it has no lactose added. (Not permitted on soft diet.)

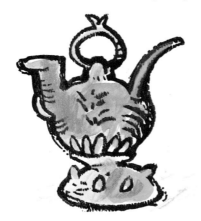

SPECIAL DIETS

Calories per SV	Protein g/SV	Full-Liquid	Soft	Low-Residue	Low-Lactose
VANILLA/MAPLE					
159	4				
MAPLE-NUT					
207-255	5-6				
COCONUT					
218	4				

Super Frozen Delight

1 package instant pudding
(chocolate, vanilla,
butterscotch, or lemon)

2 cups of chilled Isomil or
Neumullsoy
2 cups nondairy whipped
topping

Read the label of pudding mix to see that no milk or other milk product
has been included. Prepare pudding as directed, substituting Isomil or
Neomullsoy for milk. Gently fold in whipped topping. Pour into freezer
container, cover, and freeze until firm, about 3 hours. Makes 1 quart (8
servings).

Nut Delight: Fold in 1 cup of your favorite chopped nuts with the
whipped topping. (Not permitted on soft diet.)

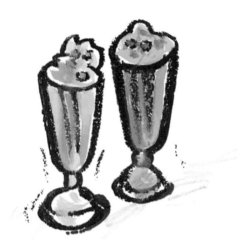

| | | SPECIAL DIETS | | | |
Calories per SV	Protein g/SV	Full-Liquid	Soft	Low-Residue	Low-Lactose
133	1				

Recipe Index